S
Cons

"Everything is connected. Consciousness is the connection. *Seeding Consciousness* helps us awaken to the interconnections of a conscious universe. It helps transcend the illusions of separateness and inertness."

VANDANA SHIVA, ENVIRONMENTAL ACTIVIST,
FOOD SOVEREIGNTY ADVOCATE, AND
AUTHOR OF *SACRED SEED*

"In today's rapidly expanding psychedelic movement, few people have taken the plunge into the mysterious, mystical, and magical waters that are the very core of what psychedelic exploration is all about. Tricia is one of these people: she is a model for others to follow and the very embodiment of the 'new thought, ancient wisdom' paradigm. *Seeding Consciousness* will not only illuminate any curiosity you have around Indigenous and ceremonial traditions, it will also inspire you to pierce the veil even further in hopes of discovering your true self. This book takes its place as a modern psychedelic classic."

ZACH LEARY, HOST OF *MAPS PODCAST* AND
AUTHOR OF *YOUR EXTRAORDINARY MIND*

"A unique contribution to the growing body of literature on psychedelics, one that emphasizes responsibility, reciprocity, and the critical importance of set and setting—not just in ceremony but in how we approach our relationship with nature. This book will inspire many to look beyond the boundaries of conventional therapy and consider the broader implications of the psychedelic renaissance. It is a timely offering that can help shape the ethical and ecological dimensions of psychedelic use in the years to come."

RICK DOBLIN, PH.D., FOUNDER AND PRESIDENT OF THE
MULTIDISCIPLINARY ASSOCIATION FOR PSYCHEDELIC STUDIES (MAPS)

"Many of us in the Western psychedelic science world have been searching for initiated teachers with integrity and a clear vision for the urgent work of the times. From the very first page, I felt trust, gratitude, and respect for Tricia Eastman and a sense of deep relief that this book has been created."

ROSALIND WATTS, CLINICAL PSYCHOLOGIST, SPEAKER, AND CREATOR OF THE PEARL PROTOCOL

"The current psychedelic renaissance in contemporary culture and modern science presents exciting opportunities for a deeper understanding of psychological healing and growth that could improve our approach to the treatment of suffering and to living together on this planet. It also presents risks that these medicines will be misunderstood. After almost 25 years of working on clinical trials that may lead to regulatory approval of psychedelics as legal medicines, I am more convinced than ever that we must also be guided by the elders' deep ancestral wisdom that Tricia Eastman so richly shares with us in *Seeding Consciousness*. We need this book."

MICHAEL MITHOEFER, MDMA RESEARCHER

"There is no fervor like the newly converted. And nowhere is that truer than in the realm of psychedelics and healing. Fortunately, Tricia Eastman has studied lineage traditions that hold generations of wisdom and has logged more laps with clients than most facilitators. Her *Seeding Consciousness* results from that collective experience and contains perspective and knowledge that are invaluable to any seeker in these realms."

JAMIE WHEAL, AUTHOR OF *RECAPTURE THE RAPTURE*

"The weaving together of psychedelics, ancestral wisdom, deep ecology, and expanding human awareness is surely the message that plant and molecule psychedelics are bringing to us. We must go beyond an over-emphasis on personal psychology into a place of collective consciousness with all of creation. *Seeding Consciousness* will aid people in finding that deeper connection."

ADELE GETTY, DIRECTOR OF LIMINA FOUNDATION

Seeding Consciousness

PLANT MEDICINE, ANCESTRAL WISDOM, AND PSYCHEDELIC INITIATION

A Sacred Planet Book

TRICIA EASTMAN

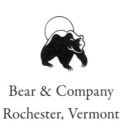

Bear & Company
Rochester, Vermont

Bear & Company
One Park Street
Rochester, Vermont 05767
www.BearandCompanyBooks.com

Bear & Company is a division of Inner Traditions International

Sacred Planet Books are curated by Richard Grossinger, Inner Traditions editorial board member and cofounder and former publisher of North Atlantic Books. The Sacred Planet collection, published under the umbrella of the Inner Traditions family of imprints, includes works on the themes of consciousness, cosmology, alternative medicine, dreams, climate, permaculture, alchemy, shamanic studies, oracles, astrology, crystals, hyperobjects, locutions, and subtle bodies.

Cataloging-in-Publication Data for this title is available from the Library of Congress

ISBN 978-1-59143-533-4 (print)
ISBN 978-1-59143-534-1 (ebook)

Printed and bound in the United States by Versa Press, Inc.

10 9 8 7 6 5 4 3 2 1

Text design and layout by Kenleigh Manseau
This book was typeset in Garamond Premier Pro with Goldenbook and Gotham used as display typefaces

To send correspondence to the author of this book, mail a first-class letter to the author c/o Inner Traditions • Bear & Company, One Park Street, Rochester, VT 05767, and we will forward the communication, or contact the author directly at **AncestralHeart.com**.

Scan the QR code and save 25% at InnerTraditions.com. Browse over 2,000 titles on spirituality, the occult, ancient mysteries, new science, holistic health, and natural medicine.

Contents

ତ৶৫

Foreword by Alex and Allyson Grey

What we love about *Seeding Consciousness* is Tricia Eastman's ability to bring an integral perspective to the complex subject of psychedelic healing. Tricia is uniquely qualified as a twenty-first-century medicine woman who has studied and embraced the world's many mystic paths and is especially alive to the foundational importance of Indigenous sacramental knowledge.

We might consider the seeds of ideas entering our consciousness every day through social media and the sometimes toxic world around us and we may wonder what is already growing in the untended garden of our minds and hearts. Tibetan Buddhist teachers have declared that certain blessed icons and artifacts can "plant a seed of liberation in the mindstream of the viewer." If cultivated, this visionary seed will grow into a tree of knowledge inside of us and bear the fruit of awakening. Whenever one has a meditative breakthrough or a psychedelic journey culminating in some unforgettable realization or a deeper understanding of the spiritual world, these mystic glimpses plant seeds for our future "liberation."

How can we nurture these spiritual epiphanies for their greatest benefit to ourselves and those around us? *Seeding Consciousness* provides many brilliant answers to this question. Tricia guides us through the lens of inner alchemy, introducing one of the best metaphors of transformation in Western Esotericism. Another chapter discusses a Japanese tradition of mending broken ceramics to help us imagine reintegrating our fragmented psyches. Experiences of ego death and rebirth are a core phenomenon of journeywork, and the author introduces some of the ways we can benefit from these distressing yet soul-revealing flashes. By providing myriad maps to integration and wholeness, from ancient Egyptian myth to Bwiti traditional knowledge, this book broadens the conversation on psychedelic healing while sharing the insights of an experienced sacramental guide. The processes of seeding consciousness and inner alchemy defined in this book lead to embodiment of the mastery template, reaching toward our highest potential as creative beings. The appendix is a treasure of Tricia's personal knowledge from working with the sacred medicine traditions of the world and cultivating alliances with wisdom keepers.

We urge you to seed your consciousness with these well-crafted approaches to the ultimate mystery of being and selfhood. You will gain a multi-perspectival understanding of the ways humanity has approached self-realization, an understanding only possible for today's psychonauts as they approach their personal Alchemical Magnum Opus of transformation and transcendence. The entire enterprise of soul renewal necessitates reorienting the greatest number of people as rapidly as possible, toward the recognition of the divinity of Nature and by fostering actions that protect and regenerate the web of life and its sacred plants in our fragile world.

ALEX AND ALLYSON GREY

Alex Grey and Allyson Grey are visionary artists renowned for their intricate, spiritually enriched paintings that explore complex themes of consciousness. Together, they founded the Chapel of Sacred Mirrors (CoSM), a center promoting spiritual and artistic development near New York City. Their collaborative efforts extend to teaching and promoting the use of art as a tool for personal and planetary awakening, making significant contributions to contemporary spiritual, psychedelic, and artistic culture.

Foreword by
Grandmother Jyoti Ma

I am proud to express my deepest appreciation for Tricia Eastman's seminal work, *Seeding Consciousness*. Through this book, she elucidates the holistic approach necessary to navigate our current era. Tricia adeptly builds a bridge between the realms of psychedelics and plant medicines, often referred to as entheogens, and the natural world cherished by the Original Caretakers of these sacred plants, who abide by age-old principles and protocols from ancient times. This book beautifully merges academic perspectives grounded in Western thought with an ancestral wisdom about the intrinsic connection to nature that has been passed down through countless generations, all united by their profound respect for Mother Earth and her vast creation. The understanding offered by this book you are holding is, I believe, essential for the ongoing evolution of consciousness and for guiding holistic healing.

I first connected with Tricia about five years ago, through my role as the convener of the International Council of Thirteen Indigenous Grandmothers. She approached me with genuine intent, wishing to amplify the endeavors of The Fountain and The Mother Earth Delegation of United Original Nations. Our collective efforts—particularly concerning the Kogi, or Kággaba Nation—have been fruitful, spiritually restoring the sacred natural sites in Colombia's Sierra Nevada de Santa Marta under the specific instructions of the Kogi *mamos*. Tricia's organization, Ancestral Heart, has been a pillar of support, funding numerous initiatives with the Kággaba Nation and The Mother Earth Delegation.

When Tricia unveiled that the medicine itself had shown her a vision instructing her to write this book, I felt compelled to support her work. Her unwavering dedication to the stewardship of these medicines and the ancestral lineages that are connected to them resonated deeply with me, in part because my own journey mirrors a lot of what is reflected in these pages. Ever since I moved to California in 1988, my life has been fully immersed in the world of entheogens. My belief is that these "medicines" seek you out. Certainly this has been true for me.

Upon relocating to California in 1988, I undertook the role of co-director at the Spiritual Emergence Network, where I would later advance to the positions of director and president of the board. I soon received an invitation to the Esalen Institute from Stan and Christina Grof. Christina envisioned a global network of individuals who had weathered spiritual emergencies. These enlightened people would guide others who were entering a broader realm of consciousness through similar pathways.

Stan and Christina helped nudge me toward my work with entheogens through an introduction to their colleague Claudio Naranjo, a psychotherapist who integrated psychotherapy with spiritual practice and psychedelics. Under their guidance, Claudio, Leo Zeff, a psychotherapist who pioneered the use of psychedelic medicines with psychotherapy, and I delved into the world of plant medicines. These plants opened and cleansed me, guiding me back to my true self. They presented a mirror, revealing facets of myself shaped by society and past traumas, facets that weren't genuinely me.

I'd been set on a path that brought me closer to the plants' Original Caretakers and their communities, which emphasized for me the importance of honoring and preserving traditional ways. Each lineage would bring us to the original territory of the plant teacher guiding us at the time. And these journeys let my colleagues and I build relationships with the Original Caretakers. We would come to know the plants where they first grew, and the plants would bring us into right relations with that part of Mother Earth, sharing the traditional and original protocols that instruct a way of life. When we humans follow these protocols, then Mother Earth is sustained and balance maintained. The Caretakers would introduce us to the original language of their territory, and the ceremonies that sustain this way of life. Yet it was the *plants'* ecological and cultural understanding that allowed us to truly receive the full instruction. This approach was much different from just taking a pill and being told what to expect by a doctor. It required a full shift in our lens of perception.

In a pivotal ceremony, Mother Earth entrusted me with her treasures, embodied in five lineages—peyote, ayahuasca, mushrooms, iboga, and Santa Maria (cannabis). She emphasized their sanctity and the importance of adhering to their traditions. As I navigated each lineage, I was drawn closer to their origins, connecting with their native lands and their traditional caretakers. This was more than just a consumption; it was a profound integration, leading to an understanding of the land, its language, its rituals, and the wisdom it offered.

Because I'd been invited through the doorway of the entheogens, I kept thinking that I would soon find that bridge of understanding that would acknowledge the Original Caretakers and their communities and offer reciprocity for the gathering of these sacred plants from their traditional territories. When people disregard or are unaware of these plants' origins, the cultural impact such unconsciousness brings is devastating, not only to the Earth's biodiversity but also to the peoples and communities that serve life here. In 2013, a small group of Indigenous elders, and I were called to a gathering in Colombia. There we learned of a new spiritual insight relating to the ancient Eagle and Condor prophecy. Originating from the Quechua and Hopi peoples, the Eagle and Condor prophecy foretells a time when Eagle (representing the technological and materialistic West) and Condor (representing the Original Peoples of the Americas) will unify together again in harmony, bringing balance and healing to the Earth. We were told that in 2026, the ending would fall into the beginning. Humanity was entering a thirteen-year cleansing process. The Kogi mamos said it was important to watch the ending as it fell down, to stay informed, but to stay focused on that which was breaking through into the New Dawn. These breakthroughs of understanding would be carried by those individuals, organizations, and movements that walked with the Original Principles of love, unity, collaboration, reciprocity, tolerance, heart, compassion, and the knowledge that all Life is sacred. Bearing this responsibility would require our full spiritual maturity and devotion to the Mother Earth.

The thirteen-year cleansing process that will culminate in 2026 is not merely a phase of destruction or obliteration—it's a purification, a shedding of the old to make way for the new. Prophecies have prepared us and now are instructing us in these times. To engage with them requires a state of deep listening.

In this era of global change, the elders convey to us that Mother Earth seeks not just purification from man-made toxins, but also evolution. This transformation, vast in its magnitude, is part of the natural rhythm of life, an ebb and flow of energy that has been present since the universe's inception. There will be repercussions to this cyclical shift, not just for Earth, but for all her inhabitants. As humanity, we're beckoned to elevate our consciousness, aligning with the Earth's evolutionary shifts. This call isn't merely about survival but about flourishing in harmony with a changing world.

For many, this call to action can be overwhelming. Yet the teachings of the plants, as conveyed by the elders and in the pages of this book, provide us with the tools and insights necessary to navigate these transformative times. They remind us that our individual experiences, while unique, weave a vast tapestry of interconnectedness. Our spiritual evolution is both a personal and collective endeavor. In essence, our journey is not just about reaching a destination but also about embracing the journey itself, understanding its purpose, and sowing the seeds of consciousness along the way. For in doing so, we are both honoring the ancient teachings and paving the path for a way of life that is imbued with love, light, and unity.

We are in a moment of change, and the Earth's rhythms and teachings are sending us urgent messages. From intensifying climate phenomena like typhoons, hurricanes, and earthquakes to the whisperings of the wind and the sacred songs of our elders, the signs are clear.

Seeding Consciousness bridges the understanding gap and sheds light on the importance of honoring the roots of this work and the ancestral wisdom exemplified by the Original Peoples' way of life. Tricia Eastman underscores the necessity of forging relations with the medicines and nature, from the perspective of a person diligently walking the path herself. When we approach this world humbly, allowing the spirit of the plants' intelligence to guide us, we restore our connection with nature. We then embark on healing ourselves, returning to a balanced way of living that recognizes all life as sacred.

In *Seeding Consciousness*, readers are taken on a journey to understand the alchemical process essential for the soul's realization. Tricia Eastman guides us on the transformative path the ego must undertake, shedding light on the mysteries of consciousness and helping us transition away from external to internal points of reference. Such a transition empowers us, enabling a departure from codependent relationships with ourselves and our culture. We learn to embrace the unknown, rooting ourselves in trust rather than fear.

The critical aspect of *Seeding Consciousness*, as I interpret it, is not merely the acknowledgment of ancient wisdom traditions, but the integration of their teachings into our daily lives; it's one thing to understand these teachings intellectually, and another to live them fully, to embody them.

Tricia has helped us remember how important it is to take our time, to take each step of this instruction in order to bring our awareness fully into the light of presence, and to honor the lineage of the medicine that has called us. She recognizes that the elders who hold these lineages need to come to know us and to authorize us before we serve the medicines to others.

Seeding Consciousness opens a path that helps us understand how we can all be part of the New Dawn that the Kogi and other Original Nations speak about. Prophecy is like medicine; it is not something you seek—it seeks you!

In this era of rapid change, the Earth and its ancient teachings call to us more urgently than ever. *Seeding Consciousness* is both a reflection of and a response to this call.

More than just a book, *Seeding Consciousness* is a transformative compass. It pushes us toward introspection and realignment with nature. By detailing the fundamental principles of Creation, Tricia offers tools grounded in time-tested wisdom. These aren't abstract teachings; they're practical strategies for enriching our lives and communities. They spotlight the systems that have bound us, guiding us toward liberation by embracing nature, balance, and interconnectedness.

Your heart recognizes this truth. It nudges you toward reconnection, urging you to walk this path with courage and commitment. Mother Earth's call is clear and resonant, and we are poised to respond. Now is the time to sow seeds of awareness and foster a luminous, unified future.

I leave you with one piece of advice, as a mother, grandmother, sister, and auntie who has walked this path for many miles: to hear spiritual instructions, you have to empty yourself and be humble. It's a terrible loss when you miss something due to an inability to listen. Be careful not to map what you hear onto what you have known before, to insert something or take something away. You will not understand with your mind. Only your heart can know the way to walk these steps. *Seeding*

Consciousness illuminates the journey ahead and is truly the medicine our souls are seeking for these pivotal times. I pray this book will cast a wide-reaching net, inspire collective effort, and further amplify the spirit of unity and collaboration.

JYOTI MA

Jyoti Ma, known as "Grandmother Vision Keeper," is a revered spiritual teacher and the spiritual director of the Center for Sacred Studies. She co-founded Kayumari with spiritual communities in America and Europe, and she founded The Fountain, an organization aimed at fostering an economy based on reciprocity and guided by Original Principles.

Acknowledgments

I want to offer my gratitude to all who have supported this book's manifestation. Back in December 2018, I was in Gabon for my third Bwiti initiation, through which I received homework from iboga: I was to write this book. Navigating this project has been a meticulous journey, especially considering the intricacies of bridging disparate worldviews. I've had to tread cautiously due to several factors: the sensitivity of the subject matter, the limitations on what I can disclose to those not initiated, and the potential legal risks. Moreover, I've been mindful of how my insights might be perceived by individuals lacking exposure to traditional knowledge systems, as any misinterpretation could lead to unintended negative consequences. I was frequently urged to share more by my agent, friends, and editors, but in some cases I had to honor my vows as an initiate of this sacred work. While writing the book, I spent a vast amount of time checking in with my elders to ensure I was presenting the sacred knowledge in a respectful and accurate way. I bow in eternal indebtedness to my elders and mentors: Atome Ribenga and my Bwiti family, Grandmother Jyoti Ma, Mamo Luis and the Kogi Kággaba of La Sierra, Malidoma Patrice Somé, Rutendo Ngara, Modesto Rivera, Atarangi Murupaenga, and Mindahi Crescencio Bastida Muñoz, Ph.D., for supporting me on my path of learning and growth. Please read the Wisdom Keepers appendix to learn more about each of these individuals. I urge you to support the work that they are doing in the world, as I know I will continue to.

I want to also pay homage to the elders of the Western psychedelic movement, who have made great contributions in consciousness research during difficult and risky times: Rick Doblin, Alex and Allyson Grey, Annie and Michael Mithoefer, Aldous and Laura Huxley, Alan Watts, Ram Dass, Stan and Brigitte Grof, Bill Richards, Amanda Feilding, Alexander and Ann Shulgin, Claudio Naranjo, Terence McKenna and Kathleen Harrison, Timothy and Rosemary Leary, Andrew Weil, James Fadiman, Leo Zeff, Howard and Norma Loftsof, and Don and Martha Rosenthal. Thank you for opening the door in the West for this next evolution of consciousness.

To Earth and Creator, thank you for providing all these plant medicines to heal us. I am grateful to the elements, the spirits, and these ancient ways of healing. As well, I want to acknowledge the sacred medicines that have brought me on this journey, whom I deeply love and am in service to: iboga, *Incilius alvarius* (syn. *Bufo alvarius*), psilocybin mushrooms, San Pedro cactus, ayahuasca, peyote, sacred tobacco, and all the ancestral knowledge systems and psychedelic medicines. I thank my Mixtec, Triqui, and Mayan ancestors. Thank you to Great-Grandma Maria and Great-Great-Grandma Jesus Ortega for carrying the medicine for our lineage so that I could discover our roots and carry it forward to today. My mother, Annette, and my grandmother Hazel Eastman are women of the Earth who instilled a good way in me: to plant seeds in the soil, take care of nature, lead by example, heal with plants and nature, and turn inward to pray when times are difficult. Thanks to your countless prayers, I think I turned out alright, and I made it through some heavy ancestral karma that we've all had to transcend.

My heart is overflowing with gratitude to the incredible women who supported me though vulnerable and unfamiliar territory during many phases of this project: Ruby Warrington, Sophia Rokhlin, and Stefanie Cohen. My agent, Doug Reil, believed in my work—thank you for putting up with my wild ideas and helping me find my way as a first-time author. I offer further thanks to my publisher, editors, and marketing team for their invaluable contributions to the creation and promotion of this book.

Most significantly, to all the beautiful people with whom I have worked closely and who have supported my work: You have filled me with awe and wonder. Thank you for your bravery in facing yourselves, and for allowing me to be your humble witness, which has given me deep inspiration in my writing of *Seeding Consciousness*. Specifically, to the ones who allowed me to anonymously share details about our work together, I take each person's privacy to heart and cherish the intimate gift of these experiences. Thank you for your generous sharing. I know these stories will provide support for so many people who are interested in venturing into this space.

Last, but certainly not least, I extend a deep and heartfelt thank you to my partner, Dr. Joseph Barsuglia, for embarking on this journey with me from its inception. It has been an incredible voyage of learning, healing, and sharing our life's work together as we cocreate spaces for this sacred endeavor. I thank Creator every day for the immense blessing of engaging in this dance of love and devotion alongside you.

Note to the Reader on the Use of Psychedelics

Please know that this book is not a substitute for professional medical advice, diagnosis, or treatment. The aim of this publication is to provide basic information to help individuals get started on the path of psychospiritual exploration. This book is not intended to encourage or endorse the use, possession, distribution, or manufacturing of any illegal substances, including psychedelics. It is also not intended as a substitute for professional advice, and readers are encouraged to consult with licensed professionals before making any decisions regarding their health, mental health, finances, or legal matters. If you are in need of support related to psychedelic experiences, you can call or text the Fireside Project's Psychedelic Support Line at 62-FIRESIDE.

Psychedelic and Plant Medicine

We are the ancestors of the future, and what we do now will have an impact.

LUISAH TEISH

The Kogi Kággaba

The Kogi Kággaba people are a community indigenous to the Sierra Nevada de Santa Marta mountains on Colombia's Caribbean coast. In Barcelona in 2018, I participated in an intimate circle with Kogi Mamo Luis and Mamo Evangelista for Holistic Visions with the Le Ceil Foundation, and I was profoundly moved by the depth of their wisdom. Their intricate cosmovision encompasses a profound understanding of ecosystem dynamics and the importance of maintaining harmony within ourselves and with nature. This was my second time meeting Mamo Luis, and it initiated a long relationship with the Kogi Kággaba, with whom I have humbly learned while supporting their mission and work through my nonprofit organization Ancestral Heart.

The Kogi people have an established order of spiritual leaders: the sanhas, who are holy women and midwives, and the mamos, who are male priests. The mamos are often chosen at birth by divination, after which they go into a dark cave. They are not able to see the light of day until they have passed different tests and divinations that demonstrate their level of awareness to ensure they've fully opened their consciousness, the intention of this initiation. This can take from nine to, in some cases, as long as twenty years. Once brought outside again, they serve the Earth by making important offerings of cotton, string, shells, sometimes even gold or raw gems that they call *pagamentos*, or payments, to maintain the balance between man and nature. The mamos carry a rich knowledge system of the entities involved in the sacred sites and the protocols of how ritual offerings are made.

The Kogi refer to the relatives of the West as "Little Brother," a title that speaks to our spiritual immaturity and lack of understanding of humans' role on this planet. The mamos believe they are the guardians of the Earth and, in recent years, have ventured off their mountain to remind their siblings that it is all of humanity's duty to be stewards of the Earth and to protect her. As they see it, non-Indigenous communities have forgotten how to live in balance with nature. This is generally not due to intent to harm; instead it results from a state of ignorance or fear that keeps us in unconscious behavioral patterns. We see this collective imbalance in the damage we've done to the planet and the spiritual dis-ease that has permeated modern life: a sense that our lives lack any meaning. And now time is running out; the Kogi say we must change our ways before it is too late.

This is where my work as a medicine woman comes in. My time studying with both the Kogi and other Indigenous elders has taught me that when we do not live according to the laws of the natural world, what is referred to as the "Original Instructions," we lose our connection to the web of life, which links all parts of Earth's interdependent and interrelated systems and provides a conduit through which the spirit world and the cosmos support and communicate with us.

Without this connection, we forget who we are, along with our responsibility to our planetary ecosystem. Our lives feel lackluster and our true needs for safety, creativity, love, and joy often go unmet. In showing us the patterns of nature and our place in the natural world, psychedelic and plant medicines are connectors and reminders of our shared essence. They plug us back into the great web, and in doing so can offer us clarity, healing, and a renewed sense of purpose in our lives. I will reveal to you in these pages a process I call seeding consciousness, the method of bringing the unconscious to our conscious awareness. The truth is that many of us have become detached from our own souls, which creates a profound separation from nature, ourselves, and each other. We peruse social media, heads bowed to our phones, or disassociate by engaging in addictive behaviors like abuse of alcohol and drugs. Technology keeps us perpetually "connected," yet rates of suicide, depression, and anxiety are rapidly rising. Many of us have forgotten, or are just rediscovering, our connection to the greater cosmic and invisible forces that shape our human experience. And all the while, animal species continue to become extinct daily. Millions of humans don't have access to basic needs: safety, clean water, clean air, or healthy food. Much of the world is at war. Our oceans, streams, and forests bear our industrial waste as corporations pollute en masse with no culpability.

In short, Western society is tragically and dangerously disconnected from the planet that holds us. In my own deep initiatic work with the Bwiti, an Equatorial African Ancestral tradition that works with iboga (*Tabernanthe iboga*), I have seen powerful visions revealing that this is not the first time in history we humans have come to this point. Historians like Graham Hancock are bringing this reality to the forefront, overturning the narratives written by colonists who ignore ancient societies like Atlantis or even Egypt. There have been other crises like the climate-related precipice we stand on now—so it's not too late to turn things around. I have seen a timeline in which all humans are stewards of Earth, being nourished by clean air and water, healthy food, and loving, supportive families and communities. For this vision to be realized, people will have to operate from the soul rather than from trauma, giving consideration to all life. As a result, the natural world will flourish, restored to its full beauty and splendor. I believe it is within our power, collectively, to shift the timeline and create a sustainable, healthy world for all life on this planet.

Stewardship of Mother Earth

Nature is not our enemy, to be raped and conquered.
Nature is ourselves, to be cherished and explored.

TERENCE MCKENNA

In this book we'll venture together on a wonderous journey of exploration and discovery, unearthing some of the mysteries of altered states of consciousness, plant medicine, and psychedelics. But first we'll delve into the importance of handling these powerful tools safely, sustainably, and with the utmost respect for their ancestral roots.

As we step into this sacred realm, we must remember to tread lightly, respecting the knowledge passed down through generations. By doing so, we'll build an inclusive psychedelic space that preserves the balance of historical perspectives. As Bwiti elder Bernadette Rebienot, one of the Thirteen Indigenous Grandmothers Council, said shortly before her passing, "Regarding transmission of power (through initiation), this is a very delicate topic because it's difficult to know the morality of the person who will receive it. Does he or she really measure the value of what will be received? Will he or she have the ability to take on this new responsibility? What will be the use of what will be given? . . . Like a torch whose flame makes it possible to light another torch, knowledge not only illuminates consciousness but also creates guardians of this consciousness, generating bearers of light, people who will ensure that this knowledge is protected, preserved and can be transmitted once again."

We collectively have a duty to support the stewardship of traditional wisdom and empower the remaining elders who carry this invaluable knowledge. By bringing attention to and elevating their voices and life's work, and respectfully supporting them, we can create a foundation for future generations to learn from and preserve these teachings.

We must strive to protect the bio-cultural heritage of Earth's Original Peoples by promoting responsible practices within the rapidly expanding landscape of psychedelics. I have deep concerns about capitalistic interests and those seeking power within the psychedelic movement, as we are still moving through the dark and must use great care in entering this space. But I have faith that if we all work together with the guidance of these elders' wisdom, we can build an expansive and diverse movement based on trust, collaboration, and shared resources. Think of this base that we are creating as the robust tree trunk and root from which each beautiful branch will be supported and nourished, and will flourish and bear fruit.

As someone who holds a public voice in this sphere, I openly acknowledge that navigating this terrain has often been challenging, and I've gained valuable insights through my own initial lack of understanding. It's a multifaceted realm that demands integrity for progress to be made.

As my elder, Grandma Jyoti Ma, convener of the International Council of Thirteen Indigenous Grandmothers, has said, these areas, such as ethics, training, reciprocity, and equitable access must be our "points of study." Rather than seeking black and white solutions, we must approach each piece of this complex puzzle with humility and curiosity, remembering that there is a human being who deserves compassion on the other side of each of these issues. Ultimately taking multiple approaches, listening to diverse voices, and embracing complexity will lead us into transformative action. We have to be comfortable with the disruptive nature of all aspects of this work—work that may require us to step into uncomfortable territory but that will lead to our transformation.

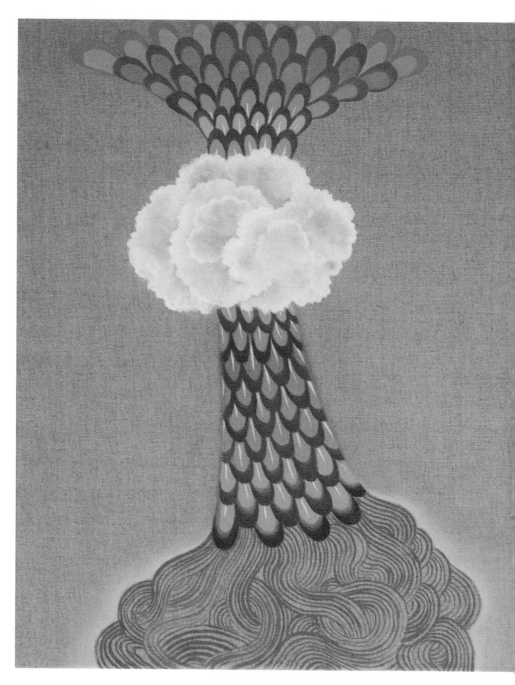

The Mystic

by Katy Lynton

1
The Web of Life
Living in Balance with Nature

*C*onsciousness, derived from the Latin roots "con," meaning "with," "together," or "jointly" and "scire," meaning "to know," originally denoted a state of shared knowledge or awareness with others called *conscientia*. This notion evolved from the Latin term *conscius*, meaning "knowing" or "aware," which stemmed from *conscire*, signifying "to be mutually aware."

However, over time, the concept of consciousness has expanded beyond mere shared knowledge or awareness. In contemporary understanding, consciousness encompasses the state of being aware of one's own existence, sensations, thoughts, and surroundings. It reflects an individual's subjective experience and perception of the world, encompassing both internal mental processes and external stimuli.

Whether looked at through the lens of modern interpretation or its ancient roots, it represents a form of unification. To reconnect with life's web, we must each use our "self" as an entry point. We must learn the art of seeding consciousness and become intimate again with our inner world. *Seeding consciousness*, as laid out in this book, refers to integrating the unconscious patterns of the psyche that create suffering and limitation and making use of ancient teachings, tools to tap into inner wisdom that can give us a deeper understanding of ourselves, our interconnectedness to all life, and the forces of nature that create change. This framework enables psychedelics and plant medicines to be used in ways that help one cultivate inner mastery through drawing from creative power while transcending the limits of the ego that lives in separation to know one's place and purpose within the great web of life.

As Chief *si?ał* (Si'ahl) of the Duwamish and Squamish peoples, who was called Seattle (Sealth), said in the Lushootseed language,

> In Native American spirituality, in Nature and in culture, seeds are the future and they are the past. They are ancestors and offspring. They are the circle of life. The Three Sisters of corn, squash, and beans were a gift from the Divine Creator, to be cherished and nurtured generation to generation. When we nurture them, they nurture us. It is a circle.
> Humankind has not woven the web of life.
> We are but one thread within it.
> Whatever we do to the web, we do to ourselves.
> All things are bound together.
> All things connect.

Just as corn, beans, and squash are inseparable sisters in Cherokee and Iroquois stories and symbolize interconnectedness and mutual support, the work of seeding our consciousness mirrors this harmonious relationship. Just as the corn provides support for the bean vines and the squash shades out weeds and preserves soil moisture, having the proper framework allows us to embrace discomfort and surrender. Similarly, just as the beans fix nitrogen in the soil, our unique gifts and new perspectives enrich the collective human experience. In both nature and consciousness, diversity and interconnection foster resilience and sustainability.

Seeding consciousness is a complex and multifaceted process. It means bringing awareness to all aspects of life by integrating new ideas, beliefs, and values into the subconscious mind to facilitate individual transformation and societal change. This germination awakens the latent gifts that live deep within all of us. This could involve the sharing of knowledge and experiences, providing guidance, or sharing stories that activate archetypal seeds hidden in the psyche. This transmission that I hope will become integrated can happen through reading this book, if you are open to receiving the seeds and tending the soil.

To "seed" our consciousness may also describe the act of planting a mental seed or intention that will grow and manifest in the physical world. Our thoughts and intentions have the power to shape the reality around us—for example, through meditation, visualization, or intention setting. Exercises are sprinkled throughout this book to engage you in this form of seeding. Moreover, since psychedelics amplify intention, a high level of awareness around this aspect of the process is essential when entering into altered states.

Finally, seeding consciousness can refer to the mystical or spiritual idea that all living beings are connected on a deep level and that by tapping into this interconnectedness, we can access higher states of consciousness and insight. This idea is found in traditions like Buddhism, Hinduism, and the ancestral knowledge systems of the Original Peoples. In this book you'll learn how to potentially gain access to this higher awareness by preparing your inner soil for mystical experiences. While mystical experiences can't be guaranteed, we can improve our chances of having them by understanding the process outlined in this book.

Ultimately, seeding consciousness starts by knowing yourself, but also being willing to let go of this preconceived understanding and step into the great unknown. It's about choosing to follow a path of wisdom encoded by Earth and trusting the fractal nature of the cosmos. It means taking choice-driven action at the right time, which is done through collecting information and doing contemplative work to test your assumptions, as well as assumptions that have been fed to you. It's how you as an organism move with nature, as a conscious being connected to the greater web of life. It is only when we learn how to work with the many layers of our psyches in concert with the cosmic forces influencing us all the time that we'll remember we, too, have a vital role to play within the greater web of life. This will bring us back into alignment with our souls and thus with our true purpose. When we operate from this place, we can tap into the source of the generative, creative power that is absolutely necessary in these times.

This book's title was inspired by my friend Alex Grey, who described to me how art has the power to plant seeds of liberation in the mindstream of the viewer and thus catalyze spiritual awakening. The Tibetan name for that which has this capability is *spongrall*, which translates as "liberation through seeing." To return to this state, our Primordial State, the essence of our being, we require transmission from one who has encountered it themselves and knows it intimately enough to communicate it through art, music, prayer, nature, story, or even architecture. The more authentic the source, the more powerful the transmission. This wisdom provides an introduction to the state of presence and awareness, known in Tibetan Buddhism as *rigpa*— the inherent nature of mind. This introduction, typically through a personal encounter, serves as a gateway to understanding. The foundational scripture of the Kar-gling Zhi-khro cycle,* a series of Tibetan Buddhist visionary practices and meditations that falls within the category of Dzogchen teachings, is named *Rig-pa Ngo-sprod*, which translates to "Introducing the Nature of Mind" or "Introduction to Awareness." In this context, "rig-pa" means the pure, innate awareness that is the true nature of the mind, and "ngo-sprod" means "introduction" or "pointing out." Through our own rig-pa, we attain a clear, unmediated perception, free from the biases and mental constructs

---

*The Kar-gling Zhi-khro cycle is closely related to the Bardo Thodol (commonly known as "The Tibetan Book of the Dead"), which also deals with deities encountered in the intermediate state between death and rebirth. giving for context and use first part or whatever feels correct to define.

that cloud our vision and authentic expression. This is the essence of the spongrall's transmission.

All the world's wisdom traditions seek to embody spiritual presence in their creative expressions and teachings. Alex Grey, who's work embodies the essence of this transmission, taking us to other worldly places, says, "Holy artworks are sacred mirrors that can transmit the highest wisdom and compassion into the heart of the beholder." We can do the same within ourselves by connecting with specific archetypes that "set us free." This is why the hero's journey and the myths of the ancients still draw us in: they unravel the stories in us and remind us to trust the sacred cycles of nature. Nature exists in this state and is in a constant meditation of these principles of living. It is the ultimate teacher.

Just as there is a mirror in sacred art, nature, and teachings, there is a mirror reflecting back to us about our inner environment. In my years of working with entheogens, studying ancient alchemical teachings, and undergoing initiations with the Bwiti people of Gabon, I have seen that the inner world—or the innerverse—is inextricably connected to the workings of the universe. And so, when we journey to our inner world, diving into the caves of our own consciousness, aiming to transform ourselves, we perform a cosmic act of healing for the wider world. Why? Because our external world is a reflection of our inner world. Thus when we are able to live as our most joyful, fully expressed selves, we become gifts to the planet, lighthouses in a world of suffering.

While it may seem audacious, individual initiation and healing can actually support global transformation. As we explore this concept, you'll see how fulfilling your deepest aspirations can contribute to others' liberation and planetary regeneration. Rather than relying solely on climate treaties or ecological summits, which often lead to temporary or unfulfilled promises, true change comes when individuals align with life's greater order. In this alignment, people naturally become stewards of the Earth, taking responsibility for our shared future. But the internal shift must precede the external shift—and I believe psychedelics and plant medicines are an essential part of this for some. I don't think it's a coincidence that there is a resurgence of so many of these ancient healing tools at a time when humanity is in such peril. Times of great upheaval allow opportunities for great growth. It looks to me like nature is supporting and preparing us to make a giant leap forward as a species if we choose to do so.

The Alchemist

Learning My Soul Name

So who am I to be positioning myself as your guide on this quest? More than anything, I see myself as a "spiritual blueprinter," someone who has studied pathways to transcendence in many different schools of ancestral wisdom. I have received insights from the plants and my initiations, which I integrate and which have started to reveal some distinctive patterns. From my collective two decades working in the wellness and psychospiritual healing space, I have discovered protocols and gathered insights into what types of blockages keep consciousness from evolving, and I've assimilated this information into a structure that can support us as we face the unique challenges of our era. I believe my superpower is creating staging processes within a longer arc of spiritual development. The question I ask is, what is the process of unfolding that seeds consciousness? These are the principles and discoveries that inform this book. Now, it is just a dip in a vast ocean of this enormous topic, but its full flowering is possible for those who commit to the process.

In 2016 I went through an initiation process into the Bwiti Fang, an esoteric wisdom school of the Bwiti people in Gabon, on the Atlantic coast of Central Africa, where I was given my official soul name. During one of these initiations, I took high doses of iboga, which is among the most potent psychoactive plants on Earth. I was directed to sit in front of a mirror, which I was told was a portal to the spirit world. The *nima*, or

Bwiti priest, instructed me and the other initiates: "You must go into the spirit world and get your *Kombo* [spiritual or initiate name]."

When I looked into the mirror, I could barely focus; my eyes wandered as if I had no control over them. Then, slowly, something started to form. I thought it was a dolphin or maybe a mermaid. My mind tried to grab hold of the image, but each time, it would vanish. Finally, after many grueling hours of practicing this meditation in the mirror under the powerful effects of the plant, an old African woman's face appeared. She spoke what sounded like the word *mboumba*, as images of a kundalini spiral and two serpents, one black and one white, birthed from her mouth and rose to the heavens. The word *mboumba* is connected to an initiation called Mboumba Eyano or Mboumba Yano, which is associated with the kundalini, the quintessence of our creative energy and used for reaching trance or mystical states.

From what I understand about the meaning of my name, she was letting me know that I embody the archetype of the alchemist. This word was my interpretation, as *alchemist* is not a word that exists in Bwiti. The nima said to me that it means "world-bridger." A person who bridges worlds might be called a shaman by some, but personally I try to only use that word sparingly in reference to this work, because it belongs to the Mongolian tradition, derived from the Russian word *sămăn*, and has been frequently misused in the Western culture as a blanket term. One of my elders, Malidoma Patrice Somé, (who passed recently) has called me a woman of medicine. Sometimes I might refer to this, as it used within my ancestral *mestiza* heritage of traditional *curanderismo* and its ritualists. It is now also a phrase that some are misappropriating.

An alchemist or world-bridger has a deep understanding of the elements that make up the universe and the transformations these elements must undergo as part of our evolutionary spiral. Paralleling this concept is a medicinal practice of inner alchemy, which is the art of conjuring harmony from discord, of transforming our suffering into gold.

This work is part of a multilayered process of seeding our consciousness and can be facilitated by the use of psychedelics—as I will be illuminating for you here. My intention is to take you on a "trip" in these pages, distilling the wisdom I have been blessed to receive through initiation and through my many years of experience as a medicine woman, as well as in my study of the alchemical and esoteric. I'll illustrate how we can begin the process of turning our base understanding of ourselves and the world into creative, expansive, and illuminating gold. You can't just take a psychedelic and expect a change in your life; I learned this in my raving days. But you can use it as a tool, consciously amplifying your own internal excavation process and healing.

Ultimately, this is my humble attempt to be a conduit and bring forth the master plants as catalysts for humanity's awakening and healing. Of course, these sacred plants and their wisdom are a transmission beyond words, too vast to be explained by any current egoic reference point or model. The true gift is the actual transmission of the knowledge through the experience itself. Yet guidance is needed to understand the transmission process and how to approach it with care and respect.

I never imagined that one day I would be sitting in front of that dusty mirror in Gabon while the root bark of a powerful psychoactive shrub swirled through my system. Or that I would end up facilitating journeys for thousands of others and developing methodologies for their proper use. But after I set out on this path, I realized I had already been walking this journey for a long time.

Rediscovering the Gifts of My Ancestors

Even as a little girl, I could see into the spirit world. This gift was part of my heritage, but it had been almost lost from my lineage, as my grandfather chose to walk away from our ancestral path. My family on my mother's side are the descendants of the ancient Aztecs, specifically the Oaxacan nations of Triqui and Mixtec in Mexico. My grandfather Richard had been raised by his Aunt Maria, who was called a *bruja* (witch) by the family, but in truth was more of a ritualist. Maria, who was born in Jalisco, Mexico, practiced Santeria, a syncretic faith combining Spanish Catholicism and the traditional Yoruba religion of West Africa, which our family had practiced for several generations.

Maria had extraordinary clairvoyant powers and used divination rituals for guidance, and my grandfather grew up around these practices. But as an adult, he rejected his upbringing and eventually became a devout Catholic. As such, my mother was raised Catholic and was taught that spirits were evil, a belief instilled during colonialization to separate Indigenous peoples from their animist and nature-based belief systems.

Yet my mother was clairvoyant, and often had precognitive visions that she believed opened the door to dark spirits and would keep her from the path of God. She passed these beliefs on to me; she was afraid of my mystical gifts and protected me from the harm she felt they might cause by banning me from anything that would further open that doorway. My mother is pure of heart and a powerful healer; she would never claim so, but I've witnessed the powers of her prayers. As with Maria Sabina or other revered curanderos of Mexico, I felt like her prayers came from a higher realm beyond her. My mother never placed expectations upon me, but instead taught me the values of service to others, humility, stewardship of nature, folk craft, and natural medicine. Whenever I had a problem, she encouraged me to go within and pray. This instilled the solid base that later allowed me to begin my work with plant medicines and psychedelics, and reconnect to my ancestral traditions.

I began experimenting with altered states of consciousness in high school. I started smoking tobacco regularly, and by age fifteen I had started going to raves and taking ecstasy. By eighteen, I worked at a psychedelic bookstore and volunteered for harm reduction at warehouse raves in Seattle. But I stopped taking MDMA and magic mushrooms, my two favorite psychedelics, in my early twenties, after my birth father attempted suicide and was diagnosed with schizophrenia and was hospitalized. His marijuana abuse had triggered his psychological breakdown, and my stepdad drilled into me that I would end up like my father if I kept using "drugs." I took heed to the warning that I could "break my brain," as there was legitimate research at the time indicating the possibility that the schizophrenia gene could be activated by drug use.

Turning away from raves and psychedelics, I focused on being responsible and building a conventional success story. By twenty-eight, I had a high-paying corporate job, a home, a seemingly perfect husband, and material wealth. Yet, this pursuit of affluence left me unsatisfied and searching for meaning in life. I was proud to have built a life for myself that lifted me out of the financial struggles that my family faced when I was growing up. But I soon realized, none of it gave me the freedom or feeling of safety I sought.

And so I started a daily yoga practice and learned how to meditate in an attempt to address this emotional and spiritual malaise. But despite marginal improvements, my trauma only seemed to amplify. I had developed social anxiety and was struggling with an eating disorder that had started in my teens. To mask the deep discomfort within me, I took Xanax during the day, drank wine before bed, and downed a venti americano coffee every morning to jump-start my tired brain. My inner turmoil left me feeling isolated and alone. I sought psychotherapy as an avenue of healing but felt it was superficial and never touched the true core of my suffering.

Finally I sought relief in the psychedelics I had once left behind. Returning to the rave scene of my youth, I found solace in wild weekends of techno-fueled dancing. I rediscovered my old friend MDMA. The drug, and the intense dancing, gave me a sense of connection to myself that I hadn't felt in a long time.

And then, on one of these wild nights, I had a mystical experience triggered by what some esoteric traditions refer to as a "kundalini awakening"—and through this experience, I made deep contact with my soul. After clubbing until the early morning hours, I took a shower and felt as if I were being bathed in white light. As the light poured down on me and the steam from the shower billowed like clouds, I heard a message: I was not living authentically or being honest with myself. After this mystical experience, it became crystal clear to me: it was time to find my true self. I also realized at that moment that this meant leaving my husband and the life we'd created together. It took some time to integrate this realization, but I knew in my heart it was the right thing to do. When I decided to walk away from my life and file for divorce at age thirty-one, my family thought I was crazy, and so did my husband. But I felt the "sanest" I had in years.

My Journey to the Sacred Medicine

Shortly after this, I began my studies with a teacher of the Ancient Mystery School traditions, and something reawakened inside me. I had decided to learn how to hone my psychic abilities by using divination tools like tarot, performing rituals, working with the Hermetic principles, and studying various forms of bioenergetic healing—many of the exact things my mother had warned me not to mess around with as a child. I also attended workshops on tantra, kundalini yoga, and meditation. During this time, I received strong signs that I felt were from my spirit guides, urging me along my journey. This helped me to make a leap of faith when, around the same time, I learned about a sacred medicine called ayahuasca and the Indigenous traditions connected to it. I hadn't sought it out, as was always my process in my journey; I let it come to me. I was invited to meet a new group of people, and the topic came up. There happened to be a traveling Colombian *taita*, a spiritual leader who holds knowledge of traditional healing practices, in town and I was invited to join the ceremony. I would never have expected that the ayahuasca I thought only existed deep in the jungle would visit me.

My first experience with the medicine had a profound effect on me. Remembering my stepfather's warnings, I asked the medicine, "Please, don't break my brain." But it did quite the opposite: it healed my noisy brain. I felt my heart opening as I connected with a profound current of self-love. Following this experience, the voices inside my brain remained quiet for a while, allowing a more authentic version of myself to peer through my cracks. The seeds of consciousness were beginning to germinate within me.

Yet something was still lacking. I felt my feelings of insecurity start to creep in. I no longer drank alcohol or took recreational and prescription drugs, but I was haunted by my eating disorders, which now seemed amplified. The torment of persistent inner criticism, comparison, feelings of unworthiness, and eating to self-soothe were back. It was as if the parts of the real world, which I had been avoiding, were clearly in front of me and the volume of my pain had been turned up. But the truth is that I had just ripped the Band-Aid off a festering wound that I now had to tend to.

At first I was filled with sorrow that the pleasant afterglow had dissipated. But I came to understand that the suffering I experienced in my mind and body during this time was pointing me toward finding the root cause of my pain. It eventually led to me learning about iboga and Bwiti, one of the oldest and most complex ancestral knowledge systems in the world. Just as ayahuasca had serendipitously shown up for me, several of my close friends were connected with iboga and ibogaine through completely different channels. One even lived in Costa Rica with a Bwiti nima. As I learned more through these various encounters. I found myself deeply drawn to this plant, even though I knew it was the Mount Everest of spiritual initiations and the most intense plant medicine of all. The draw for me was this deep-rooted feeling inside that told me iboga could free me from my eating disorders.

I had my first meeting with iboga at the Crossroads Ibogaine Treatment Center in Mexico, in the form of an extract called ibogaine. I had a healthy respect for this psychoactive medicine, as I had read that you could die from the experience if you didn't take proper precautions and follow safety protocols—which is true. The experience itself was long, scary, and uncomfortable, lasting three days. I saw the story of cosmic creation from the beginning of time and through the ages, ending in a single point of light: singularity. I was shown that this light was part of me. This understanding allowed me to detach from the idea of "self" as separate from all Creation, a belief that had made me a prisoner in my body. I saw myself from a transpersonal place, as a fractal of the entire universe. I felt like I was set free for the first time.

I cried in gratitude as what felt like eons passed after receiving this revelation. No longer confined to seeing myself as mere flesh and blood, I let go of the need for my sacred body to adhere to an unrealistic standard of perfection in order to be loved and accepted. At the end of my journey, I expressed my gratitude to the spirit of iboga for the profound blessing I'd received, and I asked, "How can I be of service to you?" Within several weeks Dr. Martin Polanco, the founder of Crossroads, invited me to work as a facilitator for the psychospiritual program at their clinic in Baja. Working alongside highly experienced doctors—who included my now-husband, psychologist and spiritual theologist Joseph Barsuglia, Ph.D.—provided a deep place of collaborative learning and growth, where our ethos was to hold each other accountable and in integrity.

Transmissions of Consciousness

Over the following nine years, I would begin my work facilitating, observing, and supporting people in their transformative experiences with iboga and other psychoactive substances, including psilocybin mushrooms and 5-MeO-DMT. Meanwhile, walking alongside me in my path was my life partner, Joseph Barsuglia, Ph.D. who had started working for MAPS as a research psychologist on the Phase II trials testing MDMA as a PTSD treatment. His expertise in neuropsychology drew him to psychedelics, as he saw that 5-MeO-DMT and ibogaine were profound tools for healing traumatic brain injury and trauma. Joseph published multiple research papers, as he also saw great potential in using both medicines to heal the effects of lifelong health issues as a result of Lyme disease. We garnered a following for our artfully curated international retreats, workshops, and events, and I received invitations to speak at conferences and on podcasts about psychedelics and plant medicines. At the core of our relationship is a pure, shared devotion to support others in spiritual growth and healing. We are always careful around the legality of the work, keeping clear boundaries around the work for retreats in varied legal jurisdictions, as it has allowed us to be more public about our work in the psychedelic space as well as advise on policy and other initiatives.

Although I knew it was risky to speak about these things, I felt a responsibility to accept these opportunities to share my experience as a woman in the space with a deep yearning to see this work flourish in society, responsibly and respectfully. My work emphasizes cultural preservation, reciprocity, and right relationship, along with holistic wellness, art, mysticism, mastery, and a high regard for the aesthetic of beauty that shows itself in the creation of harmony in our inner and outer environments. In my experience, many of these pieces are missing from the current focus of the emerging psychedelic movement, especially since capitalistic interests have flooded the space and carefully crafted experiences have been sacrificed for scalability. Sadly, many corporate forces in the movement operate in ways antithetical to central principles upheld by the ancestral stewards of these medicines, such as the primacy of nature, interconnectedness, interdependence, reciprocity, mastery of one's craft, and sharing. Now is a crucial time to be hyper-intentional about how we move forward and to protect the sacredness of this work and the vulnerability of these cultural traditions, and be sensitive to our past decades of suppression and Western attempts to wipe out Indigenous peoples.

Along the way, I have been blessed to witness profound transformations in the people I have worked with; I am enthused to share, with permission, some stories with you here. Of course, plant medicines and psychedelics are not the only paths to healing, but I now know from extensive personal experience that this path can bring deep transformation when done properly. I have also seen, time and again, that when people experience greater peace and acceptance within themselves, they become inspired to give back and be of service. They realize the human experience is not centered around taking, extracting, mining, and amassing. Instead, all things are relational; we are meant to be in reciprocity with all life. The purpose of being human is to be guardians of the Earth, just as the Kogi are. To take care of the Earth as it takes care of us. This is the right relationship.

With this book, I hope to provide powerful tools to support humanity during the window of opportunity we've been given to turn our fate around. I believe it is our destiny to evolve and transform into a beneficent, positive presence on planet Earth. It is our responsibility to find the balance that the Kogi speak of and to connect once again to the web of life. In detailing the process of seeding consciousness, my prayer is that each of us can become part of this shift.

But by no means do I claim to be a guru or an expert. I am here only to open a door and reveal a process that you must embark on within yourself—with or without the use of psychedelics and plant medicines—to discover your true quintessence. A seed represents a beginning; once planted, it must be allowed to grow into whatever is encoded within it. We can nurture it and ensure it gets the sun and nutrients it needs, but ultimately the seed's gestation relies on forces greater than us. We cannot control the weather or other stresses the vulnerable seed may endure along the way. This is where we must learn to trust. I try not to be too prescriptive for this reason. For some, engaging in this process may push the boundaries of one's comfort zone. But the answers don't always become clear until we courageously take the next step forward.

So I'm here to point you back to yourself and, perhaps most importantly, to help you build an intimate relationship of discovery within yourself in the context of your purpose in the world. This book is not meant to be an exhaustive treatise on the many schools and traditions I've studied. Instead, it is intended to share wisdom I have received through the work I've done on myself and with others over the years. In this way, I hope to challenge you to step beyond the confines of your mind. I aim to illuminate the mysterious "what" and the potent "why" of the profound alchemical process that occurs in the initiation and is induced by non-ordinary states of consciousness. This is a difficult feat, as the mystery itself is unknowable, but I provide signposts to how you can connect to the mystery for yourself. I believe these teachings can help align you with what brings you true joy, freedom, and inner peace, by building a bridge back to ancient and forgotten, yet essential, approaches to life.

Many of the traditions from which I have learned about this process, like Bwiti and Mexica, are oral traditions. They were not written down for a reason, partly because the depth and complexity they contain go beyond what can be shared with words and are experiential, to be taught through story or sometimes in the form of direct transmission from teacher to student, from generation to generation. I also want to clarify that I am not attempting to teach these traditions, only to use them to provide context and introduce new narratives for a greater understanding of the cosmos and our place within it as a species. Through reading this I believe you will connect with a primordial wisdom that endures collectively within all ancient traditions.

And like I tell everybody I work with, you may have to do some digging on your own if you want to more fully understand something I touch on here. If something calls to you, go deeper into these studies yourself. Open up, explore, and allow any wisdom that resonates to enter you.

Some of what I describe here does not come from any specific lineage. Rather the knowledge may originate from visions I've had on my medicine journeys—direct transmissions by my plant teachers—or from my experiences working with others in non-ordinary states of consciousness. Nothing you will read here is dogma; it is all offered in an attempt to help open the doors of perception. Take it, leave it, or take only what you feel resonates in your bones. It's important to me to share my understanding with as many people as possible, codifying what I've learned from the plant teachers and my experiences, as the need for this work is great right now. More and more of us are beginning to share alternate histories and teachings to those we were taught in schools and universities, and I am grateful that I was asked by the medicine to serve in this way.

Ultimately, I intend this book to offer to you a transmission of wisdom that goes beyond words, a gift that only happens when you surrender to the experience, just like with psychedelics. To receive what is being said between the lines, please allow the information to wash over you and let it trickle from your mind into your body. Commit to being okay with liminality, with not knowing the "answers." Be patient and let the process unfold, and you may begin to get a sense of the larger picture forming. Your brain is going to want to "brainify" what you read. Try to resist this urge and read with your heart instead. This can be a meditation and spiritual practice in itself, noting where the critical ego comes in and responds to unfamiliar concepts and ideas. These concepts will build and weave together at the end but will still leave a door open for you to explore the newly traversed pathways. Enter the cocoon and give yourself the space to transform. This act in itself is part of seeding your consciousness.

In a conceptual sense, this book is a mystery school, but not specific to any school or lineage; it's written to help you to enter and experience a sequence of transformation in order to help you make sense of your own inner cosmos and thus your place within the wider cosmic order, with or without psychedelics. I hope it will help you to integrate thoughts with feelings, emotions, and intuition, and reclaim your agency within your own process. By integrating all these voices, we access other realms of intelligence where our true potential and that of all humanity can be realized.

It is essential to note that this process takes dedication and regular practice. It's not easy or a shortcut; I would be doing you a disservice to tell you otherwise. Pain and suffering are a natural part of our world. But there are ways to dance through these more difficult phases in life and be resilient as they arise.

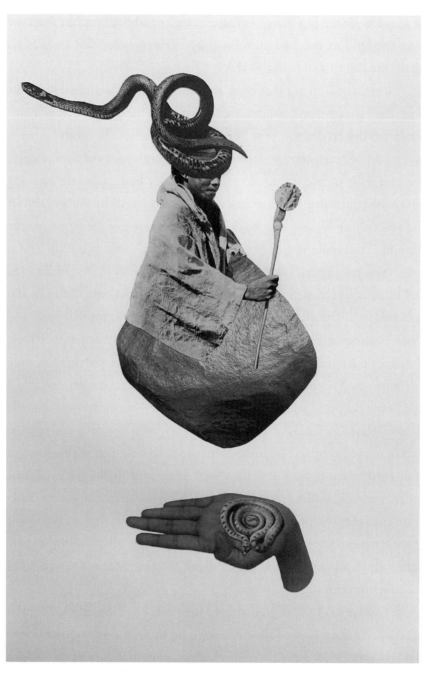

Stone Studies

by Ashley Edes

2
Seeds of Alchemy
Beginning the Great Work

*The opus alchemicum not only changes, perfects, or redeems
Nature, it also brings to perfection human existence.*

MIRCEA ELIADE

Alchemy is an ancient philosophical and proto-scientific tradition that aimed to purify, mature, and perfect. It was primarily focused on the transmutation of base metals into noble metals like gold, as well as the creation of the philosopher's stone, a legendary substance believed to grant eternal life and great wisdom. Alchemy has roots in various cultures and civilizations, such as Egypt, India, Greece, and ancient China. The complexity of alchemy arises from its multifaceted nature, as its roots integrate elements of chemistry, metallurgy, philosophy, and mysticism. It reached its zenith in medieval Europe, where alchemists synthesized knowledge from various cultures and disciplines, including Hermeticism, Gnosticism, Ayurveda, and Kabbalah.

In ancient Egypt, alchemy was practiced as both a spiritual and practical discipline, involving metallurgy, medicine, and magic. The ancient Greeks further developed alchemical concepts, incorporating philosophical ideas such as the transmutation of the soul and the search for the philosopher's stone. During the Middle Ages, alchemy flourished in Islamic and European cultures, blending scientific inquiry with mystical speculation. Alchemists sought to unravel the secrets of nature, experimenting with chemical processes, symbolic imagery, and spiritual practices in their quest for wisdom and immortality. Much of this work inspired modern day scholars such as Carl Jung. In the context of psychedelic initiation, alchemy offers a framework for understanding the profound insights and transformative experiences facilitated by entheogenic plants, linking the material and spiritual dimensions of existence in a quest for higher consciousness and self-realization.

Ancient alchemical texts are challenging to study and difficult to apply practically. Alchemists tended to write in a manner that was comprehensible primarily to their peers, rather than to the average person. They cautioned against taking their writings at face value and encouraged a deeper interpretation and understanding of the content. Alchemists often concealed their knowledge through the use of symbols and codes, veiling these higher states in philosophical and mythological allegories. This was done to keep their secrets away from the uninitiated and to protect their work from persecution, as well as to facilitate the transmission of their ideas across different cultures and languages. The enigmatic wording used in alchemical texts requires interpreters to have a deep understanding of the underlying philosophical concepts, as well as a familiarity with the symbols and their meanings. Few have the ability to read these cryptic texts and decipher their messages. Modern understanding of alchemy is so watered down that only the simplest metaphors are understood. But in fact, the power that is contained in alchemy arises when the person practicing it has done the inner work—one's internal cultivation of true power is what creates the alchemical substance.

Alchemy is deeply intertwined with spiritual and esoteric beliefs, which adds another layer of complexity to the interpretation of alchemical texts. The process of transmutation was seen as a metaphor for personal transformation and spiritual enlightenment. As such, alchemical texts often incorporate elements of mysticism, religion, and spiritual philosophy, which can be difficult to unravel and understand without a background in these disciplines. The knowledge of alchemy was often passed down through oral traditions or preserved in manuscripts that have been lost or damaged over time. This fragmentation of knowledge means that translating alchemical texts can be like trying to solve a puzzle with missing pieces.

Due to these myriad challenges, anyone attempting to interpret these works may be left with unanswered questions and unclear understandings. Yet this confusion is part of the mystical path, a first seed planted that will grow within—and it serves as an apt metaphor for the process of inner alchemy. In inner alchemy, the understanding of ourselves unfolds with time. This book will give you the chemistry set and ingredients to start the process in yourself.

Psychedelics are a natural solvent that supports the inner alchemical process. In essence, psychedelics and plant medicines clear the pathway and allow us to connect to the mystical experience which is in essence the philosopher's stone—that is, a state of being grounded in an understanding of our role within the great web of life, and of being able to hold in our minds a complex interconnected and multidimensional perspective that is ever evolving and changing. In a way, this state means turning yourself into gold. Psychedelics and plant medicines do this by quieting the ego mind, that constructed sense of "self" that we see as being separate from all that is. As we surrender to the medicine, we learn how to befriend the inner critic in the mind, or how to love the neglected inner child, or simply to receive. These plant medicines can make us aware of the warning lights on our inner dashboard that many of us have ignored or pushed away and create space to sink into our authentic selves. Inner alchemy allows us to identify, isolate, and contemplate these aspects of ourselves to move toward deeper awareness and transformation. Once reconnected to the web of life, we step out of separation and into remembering who we are and our power, while simultaneously letting go of the things we can't control. By practicing Inner alchemy, individuals can transcend limitations, heal emotional wounds, and awaken their full potential. Inner alchemy creates a fertile ground for seeding consciousness, a larger framework that can promote self-transformation, spiritual awakening, and the realization of one's true purpose.

Psychedelics and plant medicines help show us our true nature, working quickly to reveal where we have blocks and where we need to make internal changes to remove these blocks. Especially with the help of a trained and experienced guide, these tools can hold up a mirror that reflects your deeper self and where you are in your life. A psychedelic experience also opens us to other ways of looking at the world by bringing us out of our normal cognition into a state of expanded awareness, where we can see ourselves from a witness perspective. The plant medicines allow us to zoom out as we engage with separate parts of ourselves, which helps us reassemble and reorient our psyche and beliefs into a more cohesive whole, one that is more conducive to a joyful, free, and peaceful existence. All these profound uses come from understanding how to work with these tools. Inner alchemy, in essence, is a way to allow psychedelics to amplify the inner world and bring one into greater understanding of it.

Much of the stress or discomfort we experience using psychedelics occurs because they amplify our patterns, allowing us to see more clearly how we behave in the world and whether our patterns are working for us or against us. These medicines allow our perspective to zoom out or expand, showing us that we always ultimately have a choice in how we respond to life. At the same time, being confronted by difficult material or challenges in our journeys can help us in the real world when hard times come. We remember to breathe, be receptive, and let the situation play out rather than being reactive.

In fact, it is after the psychedelic initiation that the real work begins: the experience needs to be absorbed and integrated. We require time to allow the world to reflect our new framework back to us. As we respond differently to life, life responds differently to us. Often we can only understand the depth of the changes we are making on the inside by the extent to which we see the world changing. Integration can be supported through various practices, such as meditation, visualization, meaningful conversations, and connection with nature and its elements.

The recent boom in media and for-profit interest in psychedelics and plant medicines has somewhat sensationalized their superpowers. We are told that one ayahuasca journey will cure your PTSD, or three ketamine sessions will cure your depression. But the reality is that our interactions with these substances are just the beginning of the journey—a journey of learning to face yourself, to step into those liminal spaces of discomfort or darkness you'll be confronted with throughout your life, and to love and care for yourself and the world around you. It can take many years and many dances with these sacred medicines before we can unravel the false beliefs that have calcified in our beings and master our thoughts and actions in the world. It requires persistence to shed our many layers of conditioning and put the lessons we've learned into practice.

When you start on the path with psychoactive plant medicines, you enter a cycle. The process is as follows:

1. **Purge-Purify-Cleanse:** Also known as the ego death or crossing through, this stage involves releasing old patterns, beliefs, and attachments.
2. **Connection to the Numinous or Gnosis:** A direct, experiential knowledge of the ultimate reality with a newfound awareness of our interconnectedness with the cosmos, nature, our ancestors, and the elements.
3. **Integration and Rejoining Society:** It's about bringing the wisdom back into our village, transforming not just ourselves but also being in service to the world around us.

Alchemical Initiations

Alchemy is at the heart of the psychedelic experience, and ultimately it speaks to the process of transformation—the changing of one thing into something else. The practice of alchemy originated in ancient Kemet, which was Egypt's oldest recorded name. The name means "black earth." This is the rich soil called *nigredo* in alchemy, the raw material that is then alchemized into gold.

The ancient Egyptians were one of the first cultures to practice agriculture. They planted seeds in the rich soils that were left behind after the yearly flooding of the Nile, and this brought great wealth and advancements to their society. Before I venture into describing what the work of inner alchemy entails in the individual, which is the process I will be illustrating in depth in the coming pages, I'll provide a brief overview of the alchemical process to help you better understand how it can help to seed your own prosperity within the fertile soils of your psyche.

Some think of alchemy as a complex material process that turns lead into gold through chemistry. But its deeper meaning is a spiritual one: when we practice inner alchemy, we are transmuting the base or denser parts of ourselves, our conditioning and limiting beliefs (lead), into life force energy (gold). As such, the study of alchemy is the foundation of Kemetic cosmology. Some historians believe it also underlies yogic teachings, Greek mythology, and Coptic Christianity, among other mystical traditions.

In chapter 1, I explained how I was initiated into this work when I received my spiritual name. As the alchemist or world-bridger, my role is to support others on a conscious dive into the shadow parts of their psyche and help them work with these parts to bring them back into alignment with the greater whole. In the book *The Mystery of the Coniunctio*, Edward F. Edinger gleans from the work of Carl Jung that "the process of psychological differentiation is no light work; it requires the tenacity and patience of the alchemist, who must purify the body from all superfluities in the fiercest heat of the furnace." In the process of seeding consciousness, psychedelics, plant medicines, and other means of entering non-ordinary states can act as the spark that ignites this furnace.

For the alchemists of old, the goal was to be able to merge life on Earth with the divine. Like the Kogi, they understood that everything in the universe is related to everything else, and human life is both an embodiment and a reflection of the entire universe, as encapsulated in the hermetic saying: "as above, so below." This speaks to the truth of who we are: just fractals of the greater cosmological system. As such, the alchemists believed that everything in the cosmos—and therefore within us, including our physical bodies and organs and our thoughts and beliefs—is simply a different expression of the universal source energy that animates all life. Thus when we are faced with challenges as individuals, it is a sign that our connection to this energy has been severed.

And it goes further: the alchemical masters believed that the solar system's planets emit certain archetypal qualities, and that the metals found buried deep within the earth also have corresponding qualities and archetypal energies. For example, the alchemical process is based on the seven planets observable from Earth with the naked eye: the Sun, Moon, Mercury, Mars, Venus, Jupiter, and Saturn. For the alchemists, the seven known metals associated with each planet—gold, silver, mercury, iron, copper, tin, and lead—also represented different qualities of the human psyche. Within these alchemists' equations, a clearer understanding of the inner alchemical process begins to emerge, showing how transformations in our psyche correspond to transformations in the broader world and vice versa.

In some esoteric traditions, there is a belief that psychedelic plants resonate with specific metals or elements, imbuing them with spiritual qualities or energetic properties. Systems such as Ayurveda have classified plants and herbs related to their planetary connections, which all have corresponding metals, and believe in some cases that specific influences or deficiencies can be balanced through understanding how these plants can be supportive to healing. Using this principle, ayahuasca, a brew made from the *Banisteriopsis caapi* vine and *Psychotria viridis* leaves, is often associated with the element of water and the metal mercury due to its transformative and purifying effects on the psyche. Mercury is a planet of communication and ayahuasca is known to be a plant that interconnects with other plants, enhancing our abilities to communicate with them. San Pedro cactus (*Echinopsis pachanoi*), containing mescaline, is sometimes associated with the Sun (the metal gold) or Mars (the metal iron) due to its stimulating and energizing effects. It is believed to enhance courage, strength, and assertiveness. It is called the master integrator, as it has the ability to support the integration of other medicines, such as ayahuasca, due to its supportive and loving approach. Iboga is sometimes associated with Saturn or the metal lead due to its intense, introspective effects and its reputation for facilitating deep self-reflection, discipline, and personal transformation. It is the harsh teacher, like Saturn, directly and truthfully communicating. Psilocybin mushrooms are the Moon or the metal silver, which provide inner reflection and help us to dive deep into the shadows just as the mycorrhizal network composts dead plant matter to create new life.

This might all seem a little far out at this stage of our journey, but it is important that you understand the mechanisms of the alchemical process as we dive in together. Elsewhere in this book, you will learn how the energies present in the cosmos became part of you when your soul incarnated, how these energies were woven into the light of your soul and flow through your body's energy centers, or chakras. We will discover how the real magic of inner alchemy lies in learning how to work with these different energies, opening up the doors to abundance and true creative empowerment. To start, let's take a closer look at exactly how the inner alchemical process works, as this will underpin all that is to come.

The Alchemical Process

In simple forms of alchemy, there are three primary phases of transmuting a base metal to gold. These phases are known by their colors and by their Latin names—the black phase, or nigredo, the white phase, or *albedo*, and the red phase, *rubedo*. In the nigredo phase, the metal would be reduced to its barest essence before being transmuted to gold. In spiritual or inner alchemy, this phase is where we face our blocks—all the feelings and hurts we've repressed that are bumping around in our subconscious, creating chaos or disruption, and preventing our lives from flourishing. The metal lead represents the nigredo phase, the densest of all energies. In this phase, we direct the fire of our own consciousness onto the blockage, so we can distill that blockage and see it clearly. It is in the black phase that we identify the false self, or the ego, so the pure Spirit hidden within us can shine through.

During the white, or albedo, phase, we illuminate the block we've discovered by tapping into inner wisdom and asking for guidance from the spirit world to set about changing the blackened substance we revealed in the nigredo phase into a higher vibration. The albedo, represented archetypally by the Moon, is connected to the metal silver. The Moon symbolizes the soul and intuition; silver is the metal associated with reflection, connectivity, mystery, and emotions. Psychedelic medicines can be especially helpful here, as the albedo phase involves intentionally letting go, receiving guidance, and connecting with the spirit world.

In the rubedo phase, we begin working with our will to merge with our higher selves as we move through the material world. The rubedo is represented by Mars, which is associated with the energy of "action" and with the metal iron. Just like in the Iron Age, as the making of iron tools accelerated Western advancement, Mars energies help us advance today. Having identified our blocks and sought guidance from the inner source or soul, we must now act on these insights to refine the base substance of our ego into integrated spiritual wisdom. Thus the nigredo, albedo, and rubedo complete the cycles of alchemy. Now, to better understand the process, let me illustrate how I have worked with inner alchemy in my life early on.

Siddha Alchemy

When I was younger, I studied Siddha alchemy, which comes from India and is the basis for the Ayurvedic knowledge systems. Siddha alchemy was the method by which many Indian masters acquired the Siddhis, or supernatural powers, and reached enlightenment. In Siddha alchemy, metals, plants, and minerals are distilled into their essence and transformed into medicine to allow one to realize an awakened state. Mercury, the main medicine in Siddha alchemy, undergoes purification processes and is thus imbued with energies from the cosmos while the toxicity is transmuted through many phases until the mercury is safe to be ingested.* Mercury is the main medicine of Siddha alchemy because it is the communication device through which the energies from the cosmos can be delivered to us. Think of it as the conduit within the web of life.

When I began my studies, I met a Siddha alchemist named Swaha, who made *ormus*, a mystical medicine created of monoatomic elements that accelerates one's journey to enlightenment by helping one become more self-aware. As with psychedelic plant medicines, ingesting it draws our conscious awareness to previously unconscious patterns. Swaha was a businessman who chose to go to India and study the Vedic traditions after realizing he'd accumulated some negative karma by keeping a sizable sum of money from a bad business deal.

---

*Use caution and find a reputable source, as mercury is understood to be a toxin in Western medicine, which is contrary to the Siddha alchemy teachings.

He decided to donate the money to an enlightened master named Maha Siddha Ananada. Swaha did not expect to receive anything in return, but his humble gesture prompted Maha Siddha to give him a sacred alchemical treasure, *navapashanam*, as a token of gratitude. Navapashanam is a "stone" made from nine poisons that a legend says were created by an immortal alchemist by the name of Bogar, the very same teacher who appeared and taught Paramahansa Yogananda, the spiritual teacher most famous for bringing yoga to the Western world. When the navapashanam is dipped in water with prayer and intention, it creates a powerful, sacred substance that can help those who use it to manifest their heartfelt desires. It's one version of the fabled philosopher's stone.

Every full moon or solstice, Swaha invited the local community of healers, artists, and yogis to gather to make ormus. He had giant vats of water infused with the energies of the navapashanam. I, along with others, carefully stirred in Dead Sea salts and added just the right amount of lye (which evaporates out later). Recorded Vedic chants played in the background, repeating the primordial sound of Creation, "Om," while we stirred the vats with wooden sticks embedded with blessed Vedic jewels of emerald, ruby, and sapphire to infuse the energies of these stones into the ormus. As we stirred the ormus, it would attract monoatomic gold particles from the atmosphere.

Profoundly mystical things would happen through this process. During full moons or other celestial events, we would see different types of energy going into the vat of milky white ormus. The white substance would turn blue or green, or even become flecked with all the colors of the iridescent rainbow-like opal, depending on the cosmic energies present and mixed into the vat. From an inner alchemy perspective, when we stirred the vat during these full moon ormus ceremonies, we imbued the mixture with the energies of the heavens through intentional cultivation. This means tapping into the *metaphysical* mercury, the base metal of ormus, representing communication, wisdom, and the exchange of creative energies with our souls' guidance and the cosmos' energy.

As with psychedelics, applying or ingestion of these sacred alchemical substances would invoke altered states of consciousness, although much more subtle. By working with ormus, I made giant leaps on my spiritual path. I became more intuitive and connected and felt my pathways were cleared for creativity. Just like with psychedelic work, whenever I took the ormus, I set intentions for what I felt would help me move forward in my creative process. I asked for clarity on my path and for help understanding how to harness the universal energies for my personal growth in a way that aligned with my soul.

Like many of us, I immediately identified a block around money when it came to my creative self-expression, as I believed money was the primary obstacle to following the pursuits that would further my growth. This realization was in fact the nigredo, the beginning of the alchemical process followed by asking for inner guidance. Next, we need to unearth the root of anything in our path that may be blocking us from within the psyche. In alchemy, all outer changes to our lives must begin within. What I heard with the help of the ormus was, "There is some unconscious belief you hold about money that is blocking you from receiving it, and that belief is tied to the discomfort in your stomach." Using the process of inner alchemy, I had to burn away those blocks and any illusions about what money actually is.

Giving Myself Permission to Play

Growing up poor, I was teased about my clothing because I wore hand-me-downs from other families because my parents couldn't afford new ones. I got a job babysitting at age ten and started making money to buy fashionable new clothes, which I thought might stop me from being bullied. From then on, I constantly worked hard to escape my fear of being impoverished. But when I went through my divorce and went out on my own, suddenly my stability with money vanished, which was perplexing to me. I was able to amass wealth when I was married by investing in real estate, but it took me years to become financially stable again after my divorce. This is because I had set myself on the spiritual path, which activated some deep distortions within me that had to be cleared before I could operate from my authentic self. Money tends to be a sore point for many, as it ties into our belief systems around safety and being supported—our survival. As with Maslow's hierarchy of needs, we can't move towards self-actualization unless we resolve these basic survival needs first. Coming from immigrant families on both my mother and father's sides, I could see how this wound manifested.

Working with the ormus was integral to this process for me, as it opened a doorway that brought things into my consciousness that were previously hidden. I started to get curious about my blocks, and I knew I had to start excavating within. During a meditation after taking the ormus, I connected with my younger self and deeply felt all the shame I had as a poor kid, not to mention the grief from the feelings of injustice when I was bullied and the overwhelming sense of powerlessness in the situation. I saw where I had abandoned my authentic self to please others and where those patterns were still playing out in my life. I realized I had always equated poverty with being teased and bullied. I thought other kids were not kind to me during school recess, because of superficial things like what clothes I wore. As a result, I developed a belief that without money I wasn't likeable and I wouldn't be able to make friends or have fun. I thought the solution to having people like me was to have money.

I realized that, for me, money meant "permission to play and to be accepted," and no money meant no fun and not even being invited to the party. Coming to this intuitive realization was the albedo part of the inner alchemical process. Now that I thoroughly understood the unconscious patterns, it was time to move this energy to the next phase—rubedo. "What action declares the integration of this lesson?"

I asked myself. I decided to write a letter to money to express my realization and consecrate it in the material world. It said, "Money, I had you all wrong. I thought you were giving me permission to play and be accepted, which was not your role. Only I can give myself that permission. Now that I am clear, I invite you back into my life." Writing this letter was an alchemical act. I was making a declaration to reclaim my power, my gold.

To recap, my old belief that money was what gave me permission to have fun and be accepted, along with the emotions connected with that belief was the nigredo, the metal lead. The vision that I had during the meditation was the albedo: it showed me the source of my money block—being teased and feeling lonely because I was poor. By writing the letter, which was the rubedo phase, I cut the cords of my old belief system and let my subconscious know that I had brought awareness to that pattern.

Before I wrote the letter, I wasn't open to receive money because I was too busy projecting my fear onto money: that if I were broke, I wouldn't get to play, and I would feel rejection. In writing that letter, I gave myself permission to play and freed the energy that my old belief about money had locked inside me. And just after I wrote the letter, my outer world reflected back to me this inner shift. I was at Café Gratitude in Venice Beach, having lunch with friends. A guy approached us and said to me, "I have a gift for you." He handed me a crisp two-dollar bill. My jaw dropped. I told him about the letter I'd just written. Then he grabbed the bill and flipped it over, where it read, in purple stamped ink, "In pursuit of Magic." I had burned away some impurities by clearing the energy from my "money shadow," and at that moment, the universe spoke to me through this unexpected gift, showing me I had in fact opened my abundance channels.

After that, I saw an improvement in my finances, which enabled me to step more fully onto my path. The money spigot had opened again, and money flowed more readily into my life. But it wasn't because of magical thinking; it was because I had faced my fears and done the work. During this process, I became less stressed and less focused on money. The knot in my stomach had loosened. And because the knot had loosened, I could be creative and seek fulfillment in my work instead of obsessing about paying the bills. Shortly after this, I started connecting with more people who were interested in my wellness work. I wasn't making what I had been when I was married, but I was doing what I had always wanted to do, and seeing these improvements encouraged me to have faith. But I wasn't finished yet. I had many beliefs about money still to burn away, as the alchemical process goes. And I kept diving back into the nigredo as they arose. This work only accelerated when, several years later, I integrated ceremonial plant medicines into my life and practice.

The most important piece informing the inner alchemical process is the intention behind it; this helps us to gather the nigredo. We connect to the intention of what we want for ourselves or what we want to become. Then we use this intention to connect with the bigger picture in the albedo phase, collecting all the pieces that give us insight into the current place we are in. We then expand our awareness to seed our consciousness with possibilities beyond our current understanding. Tools like psychedelics or plant medicines support exploring this terrain and gathering insights. By collecting this information, we can gain clarity and burn away what is hindering us. In the rubedo part of the process, we apply our intention to take empowered action. This step can only be successful if one has gleaned enough insight to advance. Every time we set an intention, we show our willingness to focus our power on a certain area, but after we have done so, we must let go of outcomes and allow the alchemical process to take its course. Trying to control or push an agenda onto the process can fuel fear, frustration, or doubt when the results aren't as we envisioned. The way the inner alchemical process works is often counterintuitive to the conscious or rational mind. We must craft our intention, listen, and then surrender to the mystery of how the alchemical unfolding may manifest within us, through us, and around us.

· · · · · · · · · · · · · ·

SEEDING CONSCIOUSNESS IN PRACTICE

Alchemical Seeds

As we begin the journey of seeding consciousness and prepare for the process of inner alchemy that I will be guiding you through in these pages, let's start with an intentional meditation that will initiate this process within yourself.

Start by finding a comfortable seat, sitting on the floor cross-legged or in a chair. Then, connect to your breath and bring your awareness to your body.

When you feel centered, gently close your eyes and imagine you are outside in nature, holding a seed in each of your hands. These are alchemical seeds; they have the ability to be programmed with your intention. Focus on the seed in your left hand. You can put the other seed down for a moment. This left-hand seed represents the things you will receive. Take a moment to set an intention for what you want to receive while reading this book. Focus on what it would feel like for this intention to unfold in your life. Now imagine you are kneeling down on soft, rich soil. Use your left hand to plant this seed in the ground. Pat the ground with both your hands.

With your right hand pick up the second seed that you set aside. Holding this seed up to the bright Sun in your mind's eye, infuse it with an intention for this Earth and humanity. See this gift fully manifesting into fruition in your mind's eye. Kneel down again and, right next to where you planted the first seed, move aside the soft earth to create a home for your seed. Once you place it in the hole, cover it with the earth and give it a pat with both your hands. Make a commitment to tend to the seeds you've planted, as it is through consistency of practice that we see our work bear fruit.

Next, imagine you are picking up a watering can within arm's reach, and pour water delicately on both your seeds. Once the soil has been thoroughly drenched, return your focus to your breath. Feel your hands, stretch your arms and legs, and release your neck. When you feel ready, slowly open your eyes and return to the room.

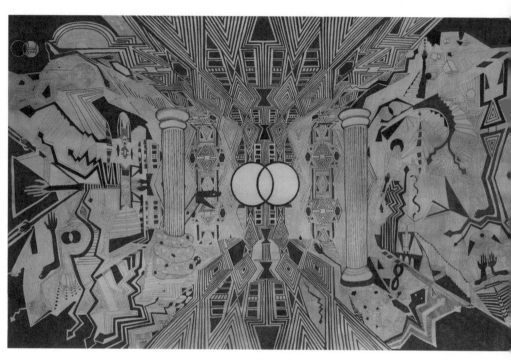

Savior Chamber

by Carly Jo Carson

3
Individuated Consciousness
Understanding the Egoic Template

Destroy your illusions so you can see reality. Destroy your fears so you can take risks. Destroy your ego so you can see life.

MAXIME LAGACÉ

To begin the work of inner alchemy, we must go inward to face our demons—like the ones I uncovered as I meditated with the ormus. When working with the nigredo, we find the courage to confront the blocks deeply calcified in the unconscious. This is where we take the fixed and unfix it. Next we connect with the albedo, finding insight to overcome these blocks by using our intuition and connecting with our ancestors, dreams, and the forces of nature. Finally, when we put what we have learned into practice, the rubedo phase of alchemy, we act from a solid connection to and understanding of our place in the web of life. To better illuminate this process, we'll explore the workings of the ego mind.

One of the foundational components of our human experience is our ego. Baba Ram Dass, a spiritual teacher, psychologist, and author of *Be Here Now* defines the ego poetically:

Your ego is a set of thoughts that define your universe.

It's like a familiar room built of thoughts; you see the universe through its windows. You are secure in it, but to the extent that you are afraid to venture outside, it has become a prison. Your ego has you conned. You believe you need its specific thoughts to survive. The ego controls you through your fear of loss of identity. To give up these thoughts, it seems, would eliminate you, so you cling to them.

There is an alternative.

You needn't destroy the ego to escape its tyranny. You can keep this familiar room to use as you wish, and you can be free to come and go. First you need to know that you are infinitely more than the ego room by which you define yourself. Once you know this, you have the power to change the ego from prison to home base.

The term "ego" refers to the psychological construct that encompasses an individual's sense of self, identity, and personal boundaries. It is the aspect of the mind that mediates between the conscious and unconscious and is responsible for managing thoughts, desires, and behaviors. The ego often seeks to maintain a favorable self-image and this can manifest in various ways, such as through pride, defensiveness, and the need for validation. The ego is where unconscious behaviors take root, and we must observe these behaviors to start the process of seeding consciousness. The negative programs in the ego are like weeds that can strangle out new seedlings that have been planted. If we pull them, they might grow right back. We must instead trace them to their roots.

Psychoactive substances can allow us to see beyond the veil of the ego, beyond limitation, and, in doing so, permit us to examine and dissolve aspects of the nigredo, or the roots of these weeds. With the help of psychedelics, we can look at wounded parts of ourselves without distaste or repulsion and see them objectively for what they are—in other words, we can engage with the nigredo. Oftentimes at the start of a psychedelic journey, we'll experience fragments of feelings, traumatic memories, or discomfort. These painful memories are calcified in the body, and the medicine brings them to the surface. Yet through this process, we gain greater access to the albedo in our daily lives, that is, the connection to our soul. Often part of the psychedelic journey itself serves as the albedo, as it allows us to receive insights from the soul and to see the bigger picture objectively. As we integrate these powerful experiences, we discover we have more fluid agency over our egoic reactions in life; we can choose love over fear, or to breathe rather than be reactive when encountering situations that would typically trigger us.

Some traditions and teachers say the ego needs to be banished altogether. But the ego is not all bad; not even close. The ego is our unique lens of perception. It just needs to be tuned and refined. As much as the ego wants to be the boss, it was never designed to run the show. For the great power of your soul held within you to be wielded, you need a vessel through which to direct it. The ego is a costume just like the body; when you strip away all the layers you are left with pure consciousness. To see past the ego and into the metaphysical realms that lie beyond the three-dimensional universe, we must first learn to separate from our egos enough to see them for what they are. When we hold the complexity of the ego and the soul, we expand in wholeness. We allow and accept rather than always *doing*. And this place of wholeness can only occur when we can create space for it all, the darkness and the light. According to psychologist Carl Jung, the transcendent function arises when an individual faces a psychological conflict or tension between two opposing forces or complexes. Through the interaction of these forces, a third, unifying element can emerge, leading to personal growth and integration. It is the psychological tension created between the two opposing forces that allows for this emergent quality. This requires conscious expansion to hold space for it all.

Without our egoic framework, we wouldn't be able to *experience* love, dancing, psychedelic states, sex, or swimming in the ocean. The ego provides a feeling of individuality. It allows each person to have a separate, unique human experience and thus to know the magic of sharing experiences with others. This separateness, however, is ultimately an illusion. In reality, all life is interconnected, and our experiences are a series of archetypal algorithms, or reoccurring story arcs that are influenced by each other and play out in each person's life. But our ego's "factory settings" typically create much suffering for us because they maintain this illusion of separation. The internal work that we do can adjust the settings, programming our ego to be less reactive, feel safer and more peaceful, and interfere with our human experience as little as possible.

What happened in the design process that made these egos so hard to deal with in the first place? To answer that question, we have to go back to our origins. Beginning in the womb and until age seven, our brain goes through a rapid development phase. A child's well-being during this period lays the groundwork for their learning, growth, and personal development. A phrase popularly attributed to the Greek philosopher Aristotle says, "Give me a child until he is seven, and I will show you the man." This blueprint stays with you throughout your entire life—unless you do the work to attune it with a new template.

Epigenetic research shows that the well-being of adult humans is dramatically shaped by the experiences of our ancestors and our interactions with our caregivers early in life. This primary relationship determines millions of neural connections that develop rapidly during the first few years of a child's life. Meanwhile studies conducted on animals at the University of Texas showed that epigenetic tags resulting from ancestral trauma are passed down, affecting the following four generations of animals.

During the formative stages of a child's development, our caretakers—usually our parents—devote much time and energy to nurturing and teaching us. As the egoic framework takes shape, those around us affirm our worthiness of love, acceptance, safety, and a feeling of being understood. But when a child is not mirrored, or "seen," by their parents or guardians during this crucial phase, a wound is created. This trauma is then encoded into the egoic template, creating suffering as we seek validation outside of ourselves and limiting our access to our power.

The Egoic Template

From the moment we enter the world, we are constantly subject to the influence of our parents, the media, societal institutions, and the culture in which we are raised. These influences shape our consciousness, creating a template—or blueprint—that determines how we experience and interact with the world. As nineteenth-century British author Samuel Smiles writes, "Childhood is like a mirror, which reflects in the afterlife the images first presented to it. The first thing continues forever with the child. The first joy, the first sorrow, the first success, the first failure, the first achievement, the first misadventure, paint the foreground of his life." Our ego typically operates from the mirrors surrounding us, for better and worse. The function of the ego is rooted in this programming, which is then superimposed onto the subconscious. The egoic template is the programming formed in our early developmental stages of childhood.

Ego allows us to function in the world, keeping us safe by warning us of hazards and governing how we relate to others. The ego has little control over our physiological functions and emotions. But it does control our ability to choose and respond to situations we find ourselves in. A great deal of our emotional suffering occurs when the egoic function gets in the way, "playing it safe" and seeking comfort and familiarity to protect us. As the existential philosopher Friedrich Nietzsche highlights, "Whenever I climb, I am followed by a dog called 'Ego.'" As we mature, this patterning becomes our subconscious mind, playing in the background to perform basic tasks like regulating breathing but also expressing feelings and responding to hazards by releasing hormones to support us.

Our egoic template is formed from our subjective perception and experiences. Outside influences or distortions from societal or ancestral conditioning hinder our ability to access our authentic power, will, or agency. We can think of these distortions as fractures that prevent our authentic and creative energy from flowing freely, potentially causing overcompensation in our interactions, which carries over into our adult years. Because the ego sees itself as separate from its creative power, it tends to exert control, seek external validation, and often is impatient.

Creative energy is the *prima materia* or "first substance" in alchemical teachings: the purest and greatest expression of our potential to manifest reality. Creativity comes through being present and open to new possibilities. When we let go of expectations based on past conditioning, we allow something greater than ourselves and what we "know" to emerge. This vulnerability, being open to what lies beyond ego, can lead us to creativity and possibility. But the ego struggles to make space for vulnerability because the egoic template is programmed to keep us safe by shying away from uncertainty. To access our real power, we must forge a connection to these hurting parts of ourselves; we need to face our fears in order to transcend them. As we build trust and start to heal this part of the psyche, we begin to lead from our soul, as we are consciously watering the seeds within to bring to flower the gifts that lie beyond the constraints of trauma.

Our incessant tendency to seek answers and validation from the outside, rather than from within ourselves, can manifest in addictive or compulsive behaviors akin to what Buddhism refers to as "hungry ghosts." This addictive patterning perpetuates the need to categorize or reduce the world around us. When we operate in this fashion, we perpetuate the self-limiting tendencies of the egoic template, and can unknowingly push away important signs, cues, or lessons. These signs can be emotions, guidance from the spirit world, insights from our soul, or receptivity to universal grace. The addictive mind, a guardian within the egoic template, immediately applies labels to sensations, emotions, thoughts, and events to insulate itself and create safety. This shield from vulnerability blocks the creative alchemical process.

This is why the Buddha said, "The root of suffering is attachment."* We take ourselves out of the present moment by obsessing over what we want in the future. This attachment affects our behavior, as we are not feeling or acting intuitively but rather making decisions that steer us toward the object of unconscious desire, without considering whether the pursuit of this object is truly in our best interest. Attachment behavior manifests in self-seeking based on our internal preferences, keeping us treading along well-worn neural pathways and often resulting in self-sabotaging habits.

Communal vs. Nuclear Families

In the family dynamics of modern industrialized societies, I have observed a notable phenomenon that differs from Indigenous cultures: the overdevelopment and imbalance of the egoic template. This imbalance has been accentuated by the constant grasping and striving fostered by the capitalist economic framework. It is this very framework that lies at the root of much of the suffering experienced by individuals, the very suffering that many seek to address through their psychedelic journeys. Where can we trace this developmental difference to?

From an evolutionary perspective, humans have lived in communal environments for longer than the nuclear arrangements of modern day. Before the dawn of industrialized, large-scale urban cities, we humans lived in smaller villages, communities, and kinship networks. Communal parenting fulfilled the mirroring needs of children, who

---

*From the Sunakkhatta Sutta (see also Latukikopama Sutta).

were attended to by not just two parental mirrors but many. Aunts, uncles, neighbors, and other children lived together, mutually supporting and reinforcing each child's safety, self-esteem, well-being, and growth. Within this communal structure emerges rituals and rites of passage that support the social and spiritual growth of younger individuals rising into adulthood.

In some Māori communities in the land of Aotearoa, now called New Zealand, there exists a recognized ritual encompassing *whanau* (family) and *hapori* (community or tribal responsibility) dedicated to a child's growth, nurturing, and well-being. Atarangi Murupaenga, a teacher of the ancestral knowledge of her lineage who was raised in the coastal community of Ahipara, shares that this practice often commences even before birth, with activities aimed at shaping the child's character and connection to their heritage.

During the pre-birth phase, songs are sung, stories are recounted, and specific types of prayer known as *takutaku* are chanted to the unborn child. These rituals are often led by the elders, who are revered for their wisdom in determining what spiritual and emotional gifts to bestow upon the child. Within the family, tribal songs carry subliminal codes that impart virtues such as strength, kindness, respect, care, honor, hard work, and honesty, and skills like oration, hunting, fishing, or gardening—depending on the child's natural inclinations.

In Māori culture, a ritual called *powhiri* is performed during the child's birthing, according to Maori wisdom keeper, Atarangi Murupaenga. It is an invocation that essentially tells the child, "The time is now. Come forth; know that you are wanted and loved. We're ready for you." This beautiful ceremony signifies the community's collective embrace, desire, and readiness to welcome the new life, setting the stage for the child's role within the tribe and reinforcing their connection to the Māori culture.

Rituals that integrate children into the community create adults who are integrated human beings. Integrated beings have seen the reflection of their worthiness of love and value within the community of aunts, uncles, elders, mothers, fathers, and peers. This need for one's existence to be validated is the basis for contentment and self-esteem in adulthood.

As the global population migrated to cities, the valuable teachings and customs for raising children rapidly declined. The erosion of community-oriented child-rearing systems in the West began with the decentralization of the community, resulting in what is now a binary parenting system—while evolving—is often limited to a nuclear family throughout much of the Western world. In the frenzied migration to cities, we lost precious connections shaping how we learn, grow, and relate to ourselves and others.

Despite the rapid pace of urbanization worldwide, some Indigenous communities continue to spend a great deal of time in villages with their elders, often living together in small societies or households. These closely knit communities are more likely to create a sense of belonging, safety, and feeling seen. Gender roles are more fluid and a diversity of expressions of gender are welcomed and accepted. Each member of the community has roles and responsibilities to care for and support each other, and some communities have established practices around how to address conflicts or disputes. Talking circles are a practice utilized in various Indigenous cultures, particularly in North America, as a method for conflict resolution, community building, and healing. The Four Worlds Institute, led by Chief Phil Lane Jr., emphasizes the significance of talking circles in Indigenous traditions, particularly through the teachings of Elders Abe Burnstick (Dakota/Cree) and Eddie Belrose (Cree), who passed on the Talking Stick Teachings in 1975 at the Sweat House Lodge in Corvallis, Oregon.

According to the guidelines provided by the Four Worlds Institute, talking circles create a safe space for sharing, listening, and exploring different points of view without criticism or judgment. By adhering to these principles, talking circles serve as a powerful tool for promoting communication, reconciliation, and healing within Indigenous communities and beyond. They embody values of respect, inclusivity, and collective wisdom, offering a constructive framework for addressing conflicts and fostering mutual understanding.

Bruce Parry, an award-winning documentarian and Indigenous rights advocate, speaks of his experiences with the Penan people in Borneo, who have a decentralized egalitarian society where power is shared equally between all, and everyone has a voice. According to Parry, the Penan have "created a society that has accentuated the traits which naturally lead to equality." In other words, this collectivism helps keep the human ego "right-size." By contrast, the more individuated, self-serving, and competitive a society, the more the egos of the individuals making up this society will swell out of proportion.

Thus the way we start to become a happier, healthier society like the Panan or the Kogi is to address the overdevelopment or imbalance of the egoic template, which stems from dualistic thinking rooted in dichotomous perceptions like good and evil, black and white, male and female. For example, rigid, dichotomous expressions of masculinity and femininity and a lack of diversity in the gender expression of role models may leave a mark of trauma etched into the egoic template. Gender roles are often learned from our parents and reiterated by society and families consisting of only a mother and father, which can create binary reasoning in their offspring. Conversely, children with diverse role models tend to evolve an integrated way of thinking. I also sense that this is why we see such shifts in gender identification in Western culture: we all need to switch to a more androgynous way of being and thinking.

Similarly, labeling certain emotions as "good" or "bad" creates polarity. Polarized views only lead to more separation and limit us from embracing complexity, perpetuating disconnection. From what I have experienced as a facilitator, it is common to see an individual reject an experience or even react to something they believe "should not be happening"—even if what they are experiencing as painful or distressing, could benefit them. These continuous patterns of rejection leave us plagued by feelings of scarcity, believing we never have enough, or we never are enough. When operating from this perspective, a person can never be truly satisfied or grateful. And so the cycle of continuous craving and grasping continues. By integrating difficult experiences, we receive wisdom and even at times can develop a sense of gratitude for what happened.

When we practice deep acceptance of the totality of our present circumstance—including our emotions, thoughts, and mindset—we begin to dissolve the barriers of "good" and "bad." The way to break down these walls and step out of compartmentalized ways of thinking is to resist the urge to judge. Sometimes our need to judge is a guardian within the egoic template that has used this strategy to keep us safe. It does this by thinking that if it can control what is accepted and rejected, it will protect you or be safe. But the reality is that you aren't any safer when you are "in control." Actually, you are less safe because your judging controller is taking up the space that should be receiving other important data input that would actually keep you safe, such as feelings and intuition. By blocking these inputs, you end up completely boxed into your head, a prison of your own making. When we assume someone's intentions without knowing the full context or backstory or make snap judgments about people's character or worth without taking the time to understand their circumstances or perspective, we close our heart to that person. By practicing mindfulness, seeking understanding, challenging assumptions, and cultivating compassion, we can gradually loosen the grip of judgment and open ourselves to a more spacious and accepting way of relating.

Our tendency to categorize everyone and everything as "good" or "bad" is ultimately a coping mechanism. This logical way of thinking can foster a sense of safety or predictability. The categorical, rational part of the brain is not always a reliable information processor on its own. Who would want the mind solely driving our human experience rather than the soul and heart? A purely rational world would be sterile, loveless, far less spontaneous, and no fun at all.

Psychedelics and plant medicines help us face the pain and fear that cause us to push things away and keep us stuck in the head, thus they allow us to connect to our inner wisdom as the voices of the egoic template subside, as they are integrated.

Attuning the Ego

Our internal and external conflicts have many causes, including generations of inherited trauma. Human beings accumulate trauma over successive generations, amassing karmic debts inherited by our offspring. Ancestral trauma is often unconsciously passed down over several generations, and it takes an act of bravery to break the cycle.

In consideration to the recognition of inherited trauma and its intergenerational impact, the cosmovision of the Kogi Kággaba encompasses a similar concept to that of karma, which they call debt. This is not the kind that you amass from loans or credit cards, but these are debts to Creator who owns everything. Everything that the Kogi borrow from Creator, the air breathed, the water drank, the food that nourishes them, must be paid for with pagamentos or offerings. The Kogi aim to end their lives "without debts" to remain in balance. This means that children will not inherit their parents' "debts;" in other words, one's trauma will not be passed down to the next generation. Everyone is responsible for resolving the debts they create in their lifetime. The Kogi Kággaba believe it is their responsibility to pay the debts to maintain their balance with nature. This way of approaching life prevents a line of suffering from repeating throughout the lineage—trauma and suffering being the shadow of the egoic template. The Kogi walk cautiously, believing the connection to Mother Earth is sacred, and that when one becomes out of balance, the connection can be lost.

We too can heal our trauma and resolve our debts, so as not to hand them down to future generations, by intentionally attuning the ego. Just as we would meticulously care for and honor a sacred heirloom entrusted to us by a revered ancestor, it is essential to approach the transmission of our ancestral legacy with reverence and mindfulness. This ancestral legacy, imbued with the weight of generations, like the sacred heirloom is an invaluable inheritance passed down through the ages. In recognizing the profound significance of this relic, we understand the responsibility bestowed upon us to safeguard and cleanse it before passing it on to future generations. Through acts of self-reflection, spiritual practice, and ancestral healing, we can purify the trauma and elevate the legacy we pass on, ensuring that future generations receive a sacred inheritance untainted by the burdens of the past. In doing so, we fulfill our sacred duty as custodians of our ancestral lineage, and of planet Earth.

This means intentionally working to integrate any exiled or rogue parts of the self that are not aligned with the quintessence of the soul— one of the core components of any psychedelic initiation. As discussed above, when we are children, these parts form the egoic template. To help us cope with our surroundings, the rebel parts of ourselves are called into action to protect us from whatever might be overwhelming to our young psyche. Like a Band-Aid on a wound, they get the job done, but eventually some real inner repair is needed to allow the bandage to come off.

For example, a people pleaser Band-Aid might have developed so you could earn love and acceptance from a mother who withheld the attention you needed as a young child. An inner critic might have formed in your psyche to get you to perform better, because your father only acknowledged you when you did well at sports or made valedictorian. These parts probably served you well at the time, ensuring your standing, safety, and connection with your family. As we mature and can take care of ourselves, the need for these parts lessens. But they are still active in the subconscious, alert for any signs of perceived danger.

As adults, these parts are likely not serving us any longer, and often make our lives more difficult as they act out in ways that can negatively impact our relationships and the world around us. Being driven by these survival-based parts can keep us small and create chaos inside, causing us to be reactive to external stimuli, which can be exhausting and prevent us from receiving information beyond trauma-based conditioning.

To make matters worse, because these rogue parts live in our subconscious, we may not even be aware that we behave in certain ways. To attune the ego, we must understand the complexities of the subconscious mind—a difficult task, as this part of the mind is largely inaccessible to us. It's what Jung called "the shadow"—the part of ourselves we either don't see or can't acknowledge. This is where psychedelics can be especially helpful. Because they tend to take our ego offline, they allow us to access our subconscious in ways we normally can't in day-to-day life.

When we see and acknowledge the wounded pieces of us and understand that they are just doing a job we asked them to do long ago, and then give them love and appreciation, they come out of the shadow and into consciousness, becoming healthily integrated into our personalities. The rogue part can be reprogrammed and accepted when we acknowledge and appreciate it, give it love, and then assign it to a different role within the psyche. Sometimes it's that simple: you can release it just by being present in that part of yourself. Other times, you might give attention to a rogue part of yourself in phases and layers, eventually allowing it to rejoin your whole self.

Journeywork

Now let me show you how this works. The methods we use in Bwiti for healing the sick parts of the ego bear some resemblance to a therapeutic technique called Internal Family Systems, developed by the American therapist Richard Schwartz in the 1980s. However the Bwiti have been using tools similar to these for hundreds, if not thousands, of years. Some aspects of this work might feel like psychomagic, a term popularized by the great Chilean film director, writer, and therapist Alejandro Jodorowsky, who said, "It is easier for the unconscious to understand dream language than rational language." Jodorowsky would often assign initiation-like rituals to his therapy clients to heal psychospiritual wounds. For instance, a patient with deep birth trauma might be required to reenact their birth. Actors would play his parents and give the "newborn" milk while holding their "baby" in a loving, nurturing way. This act would "rebirth" the person and allow his "parents" to nurture him in the way his real parents weren't able to at the time due to their own trauma.

I have witnessed individuals revert to preverbal states in psychospiritual therapy sessions, where just the act of being consciously seen by the facilitators, as surrogate parents, through being a loving witness, fulfilled a missing piece to heal a deep wounding of early infant neglect. The objective of these approaches is to mend fractures within the psyche resulting from emotional trauma. The underlying idea is that the unconscious mind interprets symbolic acts performed during rituals as real experiences. Whether it's engaging with the symbolism of the psyche in a psychedelic state, through dreamlike visions, during therapeutic sessions, or via tailored rituals, the subconscious pattern is brought into wholeness through reenactment, essentially being "tricked" into healing itself.

Journeywork doesn't follow a delineated formula. Rather, it progresses intuitively, as the traditional medicine or facilitator performing the ritual receives feedback from questions asked of the subject. It is a form of inner alchemy in the sense that it fixates on an aspect of the subconscious psyche, then transforms it through a series of questions, many of which were formulated in advance by the participant. These questions are posed so that a person's subconscious supports them in creating a healing story of realization, acceptance, closure, and transformation. It is like a detective game, getting as much information as possible by asking open-ended questions to understand where a certain part of oneself came from and what it needs. Sometimes these parts will run away or behave like children, so working with them takes patience and diligence.

During an iboga ceremony, the plant spirit of iboga interacts with the journeyers and the facilitator throughout the process. When a facilitator is supporting a journeyer, they never insert any new ideas. They simply shepherd a process and provide support for that person, helping to unravel any blocks that emerge in the form of images or symbols communicated by the subconscious mind and the medicine through the journeyer's visions. The facilitator asks questions that the journeyer has prepared in advance to dig deeper into the psyche and get clarity around important issues in their life.

You might remember the storybook *The Magic School Bus*, in which the teacher shrinks down the class and the students venture into the human body to learn about its innerworkings. Imagine if we did that right now: if we dropped through your pupil and parked the school bus in your brain, what would we see? I have done this hundreds of times in subconscious work.

So let's imagine we're inside your head having a look around. Here's how this process works:

ME: What do you see in there?

JOURNEYER: Some dusty old filing cabinets.

ME: Open the heavy drawer and pull out the first file. What does it say?

JOURNEYER: "Doubts."

ME: What's inside this file?

JOURNEYER: *[stammering]* I see my self-doubt, not believing in myself.

ME: Why do you doubt yourself?

JOURNEYER: Because I'm afraid I might fail.

ME: What do you fear in failure?"

JOURNEYER: Well, nothing, I suppose . . . I think this comes from my father's pressure for me to be successful."

ME: Is there anything else you need to know about that?

JOURNEYER: No, throw that away.

ME: Okay, do it.

[The journeyer throws the file in a trash bin with great resolve. Next they open a thick file marked "Fear."]

JOURNEYER: When I opened it up, all I could see was a giant safe.

ME: Say hello to the safe and ask what is in there.

JOURNEYER: Okay. Hello, safe. Good to see you. May I ask what's inside you?

ME: What happened?

JOURNEYER: The safe cracked the door, but then it slammed shut.

ME: Maybe let the safe know you're here to help, and ask what it needs.

JOURNEYER: I'm not here to hurt you.

[The journeyer waits for a response. The safe's door eases open again, cautiously. The journeyer realizes the safe's message is that they are safe. That feeling of safety sinks deeply within . . . The journeyer boldly throws away the overflowing "Fear" file.]

And so the cleaning continues. The stack of files thins as we pile more and more into the overflowing trash bin. It's not always that easy, however. Sometimes we must probe deeper into the files and find out why they are there before we can eliminate them. You might even need to create new files to replace the old ones, filled with your dreams, new beliefs, or lessons learned.

Is this what one might encounter in *your* brain? Each time working with an individual in the journeywork space is magically unique, but there is always lots of cleaning and excavation to do. And sometimes we run into parts of the psyche that we need to engage with before we can heal and integrate them. Let me give you an example.

Excellence Officer

An individual had come to me because he wanted to open his heart. Several hours into the journey, I could tell he was irritable and having a hard time with the medicine. I thought assisting him with some journeywork might help him relax so as to better navigate the medicine. Instructing him to close his eyes, I asked where he felt most blocked. He said his heart. So I told him to go inside his heart. Once we were in his heart, where he had many walls up, we looked around.

"What do you see?" I asked him. Sometimes, under the medicine, vivid scenes will appear and fade.

"It looks like an old, dingy, outdated diner," he said.

"I gather you might find enjoyment in caring for others and entertaining," I observed.

"So, within the diner of his heart, we concluded, 'It might be a good idea to renovate this place, make it a warmer haven for loved ones to gather.'" Whether or not there was a "real" diner in his heart or whether we were actually renovating didn't matter—either way, what was happening represented something in the psyche. He was working on an aspect of his subconscious.

The participant was opening his heart in a new capacity, making it a more inviting home. He added brighter paint and bigger windows to let in more light, until he had a fully updated restaurant filled with plants and art. Then he invited everyone he loved to celebrate the reopening of his restaurant.

Between pauses, as he did the work inside, I crouched near him and could feel the gears turning within.

"What's going on in there?" I asked.

He said, "A serious figure suddenly walked in and shut the café down."

"Who is it?"

When he asked the figure to identify himself, he learned it was the health inspector! The health inspector came to his restaurant to shut it down. I was a bit puzzled by this myself. After some further questions, we realized it was the inner critic aspect dressed up like a health inspector. Instead of kicking him out, we engaged with him. The way to reform an exiled part of ourselves is to build a positive relationship with it. This process takes time and patience—usually these characters are suspicious of any games or techniques.

I suggested, "Maybe ask him if you can have a meeting with him." There was a long pause again; then I said, "What happened?"

"He took me to his office," the participant said.

"What does it look like?"

"Dingy, dark. There's a big, clunky old desk."

I suggested he start by telling the inspector that "we know he's working really hard in service to you, and you'd like to offer him a promotion." I wanted the inner critic to know that we valued his dedication to his role. After all, the inner critic was doing the job the participant had enlisted him to do, probably as a kid, to keep him safe. I wanted this unloved and hardworking part of my patient to know it was appreciated, which I sensed would calm it down and stop it acting out so much.

My participant concluded that he would promote the inner critic to Excellence Officer, to recognize his efforts so they could both be on the same team. He even gave the critic a beautiful penthouse office *with a coastal view. He adorned the office with a red velvet couch, indoor plants, and a gleaming wooden desk. The participant picked out some art he thought the Excellence Officer would like. This was the kind of office meant for a highly regarded advisor. Once the Excellence Officer was happy with his office, we gave him a new job description. From now on, rather than comparing my participant to other people, as he usually did, the excellence officer was only allowed to compare him to former versions of himself and to point out areas for growth and improvement in a positive way. The critic agreed, and we set him free to start in his new position.*

In the following days, I sensed a struggle going on within my participant's mind. Maybe his brain was trying to make sense of it all. Maybe the inner critic needed clarification about whether he really had gotten a promotion. I told him that this can happen during the integration process, when the ego tries to grasp something beyond this world.

The following day, he was mulling over what I'd said and was feeling better. He had taken a step toward accepting the mysterious parts of himself and connecting with the symbolic or archetypal mind, whether or not his conscious mind could understand it. Something had started to land within him; a new neural pathway had been seeded, adding a new dimension to his way of being in the world and his interactions with his psyche. His heart had begun to soften as the rigidity of his old ways eased and new forms took root.

There is a limitless cast of characters inside us. The people pleaser, the trickster, and the martyr are a few common ones I've encountered. They are parts of ourselves that we cast to play a role in our internal narrative. The ego created these characters to compensate for and protect a deep wound inside you. None of them are "bad"; all these parts need to be seen, loved, and appreciated. Once they've learned to trust you, they will begin to behave in ways that are more in alignment with your true values.

. . . .

SEEDING CONSCIOUSNESS IN PRACTICE

Bringing Your Alter Ego into Alignment

Feel free to follow the examples below, weaving in the wording that feels authentic to you.

The People Pleaser

Say to your subpersonality, "Dear People Pleaser, I appreciate your desire to keep harmony and make others happy, but it's important to prioritize our own needs too. Let's work together to find a balance where we can be compassionate toward others while also honoring our own boundaries."

Instead of constantly seeking validation from others, the people pleaser could be encouraged to prioritize self-care and assertiveness. They could take on the role of a compassionate advocate for themselves and others, standing up for what they believe in without sacrificing their own well-being.

The Trickster

Say to the subpersonality, "Trickster, I know you enjoy pushing boundaries and finding humor in unexpected situations, but sometimes your antics can cause harm or disrupt harmony. You may be using your power to avoid vulnerability or being truly honest with yourself. Let's channel your creativity and wit into constructive endeavors that bring joy without causing chaos."

The Trickster could be assigned the role of a creative problem-solver or innovator, using their quick thinking and resourcefulness to find unique solutions to challenges. They could also become a source of light-heartedness and playfulness in situations where it's appropriate.

The Martyr

Say to the subpersonality, "Martyr, your willingness to sacrifice yourself for others is admirable, but it's essential to remember that self-care is not selfish. Let's explore ways to fulfill our responsibilities without neglecting our own well-being."

Instead of constantly sacrificing their own needs for others, the Martyr could be encouraged to prioritize self-compassion and self-care.

They could become a nurturing caregiver who supports others from a place of strength and resilience, rather than depletion.

This all may sound sort of insane to you—talking to different parts of yourself, asking what they need, maybe giving them a new job description like we did with the Excellence Officer. By engaging in compassionate dialogue with these internal characters and developing new roles aligned with our true values, we can foster greater harmony and integration within ourselves. This process allows us to acknowledge and appreciate all parts of ourselves, leading to a more authentic expression of ourselves.

More often than not, our inner voice, or voices, are guiding us. How often do you hear the encouraging, "You've got this"? Or do you have an inner voice that says, "I hope I don't screw this up"? By diving into these subconscious parts, we gain deeper access to unconscious motivations that can sabotage our success. Some of these patterns and expressions have an obvious source, while others are so deeply hidden that it takes repetitive digging and integration to see relief of symptoms or changes in behavior. We must sift through and question everything happening within to bring awareness to our patterns and processes.

· · · · · · · · · · · · · ·

SEEDING CONSCIOUSNESS IN PRACTICE
Accessing the Inner Self

Planting seeds in the subconscious starts by entering a deeply relaxed yet attentive state and connecting with your psyche.

Once you find yourself in a relaxed, meditative state, imagine inviting a part of yourself to communicate with you, such as your inner critic or inner child. Start by reminding this part that you love and appreciate it. Visualize yourself standing before it. You might apologize for your shortcomings in the past and let it know you're here now. Ask it to tell you or show you what it needs. Let it know what you need in return. Pay attention to any emotions you feel when you ask questions or make a request, as this is one method by which it may communicate with you. Thank this part of yourself for its service; you might even see yourself hugging it. Let it know you are there for it and will come back to connect again.

Don't be discouraged if it doesn't happen immediately. The intentional engagement with your psyche is in some way planting the seeds, whether or not you see or feel anything. Over time, this will build a relationship with these parts of yourself, to the point that they no longer feel a need to "act out" in your daily life. When these aspects of the psyche show up, think of them as a warning light alerting you to an empty gas tank. It's simply a sign you need to fill yourself up with love, attention, or validation.

Our psyches are incredibly complex and sophisticated. In our modern, outwardly focused culture, we don't spend enough time working to build a connection with them, let alone learning to listen to what they need. Next time something comes up, try to connect with where it might be in your body, or whether it's tied to an aspect of the self like the wounded child or inner critic. Take some time to get to know this part of yourself and ask what it needs.

It is always within your power to welcome and sit with these parts. Remember, they carry clues to whatever is creating your blockages or suffering. Every creative block and every stagnation in our lives stems from a part of the egoic template that wants to be heard. What if we chose to reclaim our power by connecting to these parts and truly listening to what they have to say?

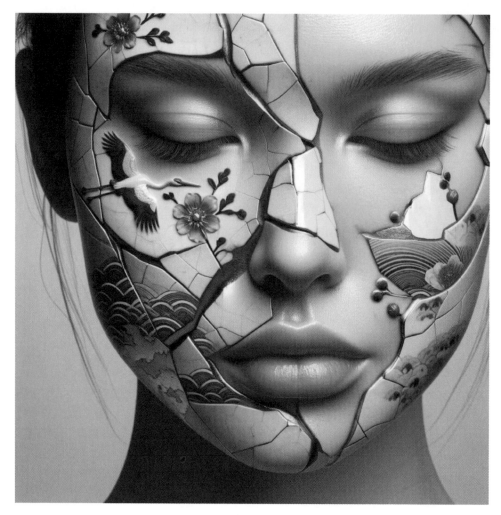

Soul Kintsugi

by Tricia Eastman

4
Soul Kintsugi
The Art of Soul Repair

I am looking forward to getting shattered only to add further elegance to myself.

AURA TREVORTNI

The process of attuning the ego described in the previous chapter paves the way for a deeper undertaking that can be thought of as "soul reclamation." A beautiful metaphor for this is found in the Japanese art of *kintsugi*, meaning golden joinery, also referred to as *kintsukuroi*, which translates as "golden repair." Thought to be at least five hundred years old, this practice involves taking pieces of broken ceramics and gluing them back together with molten gold, making the once-broken items more valuable than before they were broken. The wisdom of kintsugi can be used as a metaphor for aspects of ourselves that may seem broken or out-of-sorts and need rejoining. Putting gold on those pieces, using creativity to mend our inner fragmentation and separation, can help craft a richer and more resilient container that will emerge and ultimately flourish.

In the pantheon of ancient Kemet (ancient Egypt), the gods held in the highest regard were Isis (Auset) and her husband Osiris (Ausar). Osiris's brother Set overtook the throne by murdering his brother, cutting him into pieces, and dispersing them far and wide across the land of Kemet. Isis was summoned to recover the scattered pieces of Osiris. She assembled the pieces of her husband and resurrected him using her magic as a high priestess of the mystery school traditions. Isis brought Osiris back long enough to acquire his seed and give birth to their son Horus, who reigned as the king of the living. Osiris's mythic parable symbolizes human death, resurrection, and rebirth. As such, Isis is also known as the goddess of soul retrieval—her mythology is symbolic of the work to reclaim the parts of one's psyche that have been severed or exiled. This reclamation is the art of soul kintsugi.

These sacred initiations bring us through the difficulties of chaos and trauma back into wholeness. Yet from the Western perspective, we go to therapists or psychiatrists when we feel depressed, anxious, or have insomnia. We may be prescribed a pill that will supposedly "cure" our maladies. Western medicine has created a complex catalog of illnesses to describe these disorders. Modern medicine dissects us, leaves the pieces barely clinging together, at least on the surface, and numbs the pain— until the medication wears off. But in many ancient cultures, all these numerous labels and conditions have but one cause: *disconnection from the soul*. In fact, the Bwiti believe the root of mental illness and all emotional and spiritual dis-ease stem from a schism with the soul. These breaks or fractures leave the psyche confused and put the individual in an anxious state, yearning for the connection to one's soul that has either been lost or damaged. Without the wisdom that can only come from our souls, we can live adrift and confused.

Our society rarely acknowledges or even nurtures our connection to the soul. If you have a hard time experiencing joy, being creative, or feeling as though your life has a sense of meaning, you might be experiencing some level of schism of the soul. As such, the process of soul retrieval, or soul kintsugi, can play a significant role in curing the malaise of the Western colonized mind. In this process, the initiatic rites accompanying the work with psychedelics and plant medicines become the opening for the magical glue used to reassemble oneself into something that in its imperfectness carries even more value. Even the most fractured soul can be resurrected! The real beauty of this art is that it makes no attempt to hide any of the flaws; instead, once healed, they become the treasure itself.

From what I have learned of the soul as expressed in the cosmovision of the Kogi Kággaba, the Bwiti, the Mexica, and the Kemetic Mysteries, it would appear that many of us in the West are separated from our souls. This stems from a collective wounding rooted in the belief of separation from the spirit world and overreliance on the material world. Even for many children, society puts a damper on imaginations and tells us what is "real" or not "real." Why is it that we teach children about animism through giving life to *Thomas the Train* or baby sharks or personifying their favorite stuffed toy? Or about traditional practices such as Siberian shamanism through Santa Claus or the fairies and elementals with the tooth fairy? Then as adults we are told to discard these "make believe" ideas. This separation is imprinted on us by religion, science, and industrialization and is reinforced through our overidentification with the rational mind. What happens to the questions that lead to discoveries far outside the bounds of common societal thinking? Maybe these questions are necessary as part of exploration and discovery.

Maybe our dreams of mermaids, aliens, unicorns, fairies, and dragons give us creative power within our inner cosmos, which helps shape how we see and approach the "real" world. Our reductionist views come from scientific and logic-based thinking and have created false belief systems that dismiss the interconnectedness of life or the spiritual side of reality. We engage in structures designed and guided by the egoic template that extracts what is regarded as valuable or useful from life while discarding the rest as waste. Societies turn away from the laws of nature and instead respond from thousands of years of amassed intergenerational trauma and scarcity mindsets in Western culture. Through our extractive behaviors, we throw away many vital raw materials that nature composts to create new life. Meanwhile the false belief that the material world is the only relevant world keeps us in a restricted realm of possibilities and choices—creating a self-fulfilling prophecy of lack, pain, suffering, and fear. This, again, is the realm of the ego.

As we paint the gold to bond the broken pieces of our society, we create a vessel for the seeds of consciousness that we are nurturing within ourselves. How can we cultivate and accumulate energy that will feed the growth of our consciousness if we are filled with cracks, leaks, and holes? The alchemical gift of this process is that we create a new self out of the old.

My Initiation

I experienced soul kintsugi for myself during my first Bwiti initiation in Gabon. It took me years of studying within the Bwiti tradition to find the right village and a nima (healer) who could initiate me in a way that was safe for Westerners. Stories of deaths, malaria, animal sacrifice, blood rituals, Bwiti healers or ritualists with poor sexual boundaries, and many other complications around safety caused me to take my time. Although I had done several prior initiations outside of Gabon, some Bwitis believe only those done in Gabon are authentic. Gabon is no joke; it is jungle, unforgiving and with no creature comforts, difficult outside of even the initiation itself. When I was invited to this particular initiation, however, I could feel in my body that it was my time to go. I will share some general details about this process; however, I have been cautioned by my elders to preserve the secrecy of certain elements to protect the sacredness of the initiation.

Before I arrived in Gabon, the nima used divination to determine if I was ready to be initiated and which initiations I would be prescribed. He told me it wasn't yet the right time, but the ancestors had said it would be in a few months. Divination serves as a protection for the initiate. If they rush into the process without the proper consultations, they will not have the same spiritual protections and could fall ill or encounter some misfortune as a result. It's a blessing from the ancestors when one receives the "yes." This approach helped me to trust that I was making the right decision. Several months later, when I again checked in with the nima, he finally gave me the green light to come to Gabon.

When I arrived I was told that, as part of my initiation, I would be in a chamber for several days. When I say "chamber," I am not speaking of a beautifully decorated ritualistic space. I was led to an empty, portable structure built of tin and wood, held up on concrete blocks. But outside appearances didn't matter; the work I was doing was inside myself. The Bwiti nimas consecrate each chamber with a distinctive charge of energy that opens a pathway for teaching a particular initiation. These chambers are doorways into the schools of the higher realms. They are portals into different levels of consciousness.

I could not clearly determine the theme when I entered the chamber, but the school seemed to peer inside me, speaking to me in a way only I could understand. I was locked in this room for seven days without windows or light. I had nothing but a notebook and a pen. These rooms are much like the chambers inside the Great Pyramid of Giza in Egypt, which are also nothing but large rooms imbued with unique energies. In Egypt, each chamber "school" had a specialized teaching based on the principles of Kemetic Mystery School traditions. The branch of the Bwiti I was working with, the Fang, base their teachings on Kemetic alchemy, and they believe they were at one time connected to the people of Kemet and the pharaohs. The Bwiti father of the village who initiated me knew inherently that his tribe was from the Osirian Temple in Egypt. I saw drawings of plants in the Egyptian temples that look a lot like iboga, and the priestess Seshat wears animal skin just like the *nganga* in Bwiti. As well, it is common knowledge in Gabon that the Bwiti harpists played in the high courts of the pharaohs.

I was instructed to carry a kerosene lantern everywhere I went and to keep it close beside my bed throughout the night, to help guide me in the visionary realm. This lantern represents the initiate's soul and is a symbolic reminder always to remain connected to your soul. If I forgot my lantern, I had forgotten my soul. I could leave the chamber only to take a ritual bath with sacred plants and clays, to use the bathroom, or for my two meals a day, which I cooked in a makeshift kitchen attached to the chamber.

After three days of ritual baths, the nima came in and performed additional rituals to open the ceremonial space. Then he handed me a tall glass of tea made of iboga root bark. I was more accustomed to taking the dry, chalky brambles of shaved root bark, and I had never taken iboga in this form before. It was very bitter and numbed my throat as I tried to swallow it. Once you have tasted iboga, it almost immediately triggers a gag reflex; it is one of the most bitter things you will ever taste.

The nima spoke to me in French and, seeing that I didn't understand, he communicated with a grunt, tipping the glass to get the liquid down my throat faster. After I'd drunk the whole glassful, I signaled for some water to wash it down. The nima wouldn't give me any. My sense was that this was because it was so strong that drinking more liquid could have induced me to purge the medicine.

Seeing the unintentional contortion of my face, he must have taken pity on me, because he picked up a lollipop from the altar that was intended as an offering to the spirits, unwrapped it, and put it in my mouth in a moment of grace.

The onset of the medicine hit me really fast; less than thirty minutes passed before the room started to spin and I felt the pressure increasing in my head. I tend to be very responsive and sensitive to the medicine. My ears started buzzing and waves of heat rushed over my body. I heard a whirring sound and a spinning portal appeared above my head—then pulled me in.

I felt the familiar sensation of dropping into the spirit world, which I had experienced in past work with iboga—a sense of release akin to popping through the birth canal, as the pressure and intense spinning subsided in a sign of relief. Intense joy and gratitude filled me as I returned to these familiar sacred realms. I always feel like I've entered the backstage rooms of the universe when I sojourn with iboga. It was like a video game, as if I were interfacing with the very knobs and levers that controlled the entire cosmos. I've never felt anything grander than this passage into the ashrams of consciousness, the schools of the higher realms where you can download lifetimes of wisdom in seconds. There were chambers or spiritual classrooms where you could learn any kind of music, art, or wisdom teaching that inspired you. The great masters and creative geniuses visited these schools: Einstein, Beethoven, Hilma Klint, Yogananda, and Plato. Yet again, I was overcome with awe by the magnificence of the universe. What a creation!

At one point in the journey, an image of my soul appeared to me, bringing with it information that allowed me to use my soul as a vessel for creativity. The writing of this book, in fact, was given to me as an assignment during this initiation. Every chapter was clearly laid out for me, and I was told that writing it was a key piece of my soul's purpose. As I finished the manuscript many years later, I understood why this was my integration homework. The obstacles that came up in writing this book were more complex than the initiation itself. My inner critic taunted me many times. I had to overcome massive resistance and judgment in my writing. As a child, I'd been diagnosed with ADHD, but I learned later in adulthood that I was more neurodivergent than I had realized. Although plant medicines have helped me a great deal in my healing process, I still often struggle to articulate what I want to say, and writing an entire book was new territory for me, challenging what I know, my process, and how I communicate. I've had to destroy and rebuild some of my old coping mechanisms—and *this* was the real work for me. The truth of all initiations is that the path does not get easier; the medicine calls for an ever-deepening refinement of how we move in the world as we discover how to lean into the shadow rather than avoid it. The ego is masterful when it comes to finding ways to distract, self-soothe, or just straight up run away from what we have to face. Sometimes, it feels like the pieces of the broken vessel that need to be rejoined are like magnets repelling one another. But we have to keep patiently moving them closer together.

Soul Connections

My initiation gave me the ability to understand more clearly what my soul is and to see how separating from my soul had disempowered me in certain areas of my life. It allowed me to see the events that made me hold on to shame and low self-worth. Many of these events related to this neurodivergent part of myself that, at times, made me feel broken or powerless. What happened in the initiation chamber, some of which I can't even be sure of myself, allowed me to begin to repair this schism with my soul so I could refine my inner alchemical process, the process of soul kintsugi that was bringing these hurts into the light and inviting me to step beyond the ego constraints that kept me small and stuck.

For some individuals who approach this process, encountering the soul through iboga visions is not what they may have imagined or expected. In these visionary realms, the soul can appear as a character, a gesture, a color, or a shape. Its form may come as a surprise. We often have preconceived notions of the spirit world, sometimes based on Hollywood portrayals of these realms. From my experiences supporting others in this process, I've heard some interesting stories about what initiates saw when they first met their souls. One initiate saw his soul as a superhero with a cape and a unique symbol on his chest. Another initiate's soul was an

Egyptian pharaoh with a headdress. These costume visions are of particular significance because, in this lineage of initiation, an initiate can go to a traditional Gabonese tailor and have a costume made of their soul, which they wear in all future ceremonies and village rituals.

Once the initiate meets their soul and receives a soul name, they use that name for all future ceremonies and will no longer be called a *banzi* (which means to hatch). In the journey to find a soul name, initiates often go through experiences that don't make sense, and see imagery that's bizarre or confusing. I call this part of the journey the "soul car wash" because it's when old patterns are cleansed and purged. While you might see something of significance during this stage, such as visionary communications about your gifts, purpose, and intentions, you'll mainly be clearing the path for trudging through the realms of your unconscious mind.

On the journey, you will meet different characters. Some might be scary looking, and some divine. When they approach you, ask them, "Are you my soul?" or "What is the name of my soul?" The secret is that if you get an answer you're unsure about, it is most likely not your name. When your name is said, you'll feel it resonate in every cell of your body as truth. You will not question it. Our soul names are pivotal in initiations: they have special meanings and can reveal to us our unique spiritual identity, purpose, and gifts. The nima will have insight into the significance of the soul name, even if you do not understand what it means.

These initiation rituals are an essential part of Bwiti culture. Many cultures have similar ways to induce mystical states, some Indigenous peoples of North America practice vision quests, and some Aboriginal and Torres Strait Islander peoples have walkabout traditions that can serve as rites of passage. Some Indigenous cultures incorporate periods of solitude and challenging conditions as part of traditional practices that may facilitate profound experiences for young people transitioning into adulthood. To join the society as an adult, you must first experience the death of the ego and connect to your own soul to know your true self. The Bwiti and other Indigenous cultures mentioned above believe that to have a healthy society, each person must at some level be able to answer the question, "who am I?"

As for rites of passage in the West, our milestones often revolve around life events and societal achievements, such as getting married, having a child, or graduating college. However, unlike traditional societies with structured rituals, our culture lacks significant rites of passage and initiations guided by wise elders and this absence leaves many individuals adrift in areas of their life, still clinging to childhood behaviors and unaware of their unique roles and gifts that contribute to society.

Engaging in self-reflection can be daunting, as it often brings forth pain, discomfort, and darkness—the metaphorical tar pit or abyss that many fear confronting. Yet, as illustrated by the practice of soul kintsugi, this process is transformative. Just as crude petroleum undergoes refinement to produce massive amounts of energy, delving into our deepest wounds and shadows can unlock profound growth and creativity.

Mending the Schism of the Soul

During a soul retrieval, a traditional medicine practitioner or guide travels to the psyche or subconscious with the journeyer to help find the missing pieces of the soul, collect wisdom from them to allow one to integrate them back into the person's psyche. Once these pieces have been found and restored, the person must engage with their soul and build a relationship with it to better understand how to remain connected with it going forward. Contrary to Western wisdom, which often seeks to avoid pain at all costs, those of us who aim to reconnect to broken parts of ourselves must run *toward* our pain and give it attention and love. Love is the metaphorical "gold," the light and beauty present after each piece is glued back in place one at a time. This mending may take multiple journeys, as we must be careful to let the glue set before rushing on to the next piece.

When I work with individuals on my retreats, I support others in this process. Similar to the work with the health inspector/inner critic detailed in chapter 3, this type of soul retrieval involves diving into the psyche and asking the right questions with the aim of reconnecting with the soul.

Every psyche has its own complexities. Before starting the journey, I ask the person if they would like to engage with their soul, and to write down questions they'd like to ask of their soul. We work on the questions together in preparation, during a one-on-one interview conducted before the journeywork. Iboga appreciates precision and can offer answers more easily when provided with clear questions and intentions. During the journey, the participant lies on a bed. I tell them to leave the page of questions beside the bed, so that at some point in the journeying process I can read it to them. I let them know this will be a journey into their psyche and that they can use their imagination along with the medicine—that the imagination is an important tool for connecting with their soul and the subconscious.

A psychospiritual iboga retreat format is usually a week or longer, but two nights are dedicated to ceremony. The first ceremony night is often understood as a type of death process, and the second is rebirth. On the first night, the individual is cleansed of all that needs to be let go. A lot of purging can occur during this night. For many, this process can continue into the second night as well. But for some, who are ready, the second night is the rebirth phase of the journey, when they connect to their souls.

I can tell where each journeyer is in the process through various means—for example, by asking them what kinds of visions they're seeing, or noticing how they are walking when I help them to the bathroom. I check on them throughout, asking them how they feel and gauging where they are in the experience.

When I sense the journeyer is deep enough in the medicine, I ask if they want to go through their questions. If they agree, I tell them I will read the questions aloud and have the person verbally repeat them to their soul. The spirit of iboga works through call and response, and you will notice this in the songs the men and women sing in the villages. This format of hearing and repeating back is very important for the orientation of the journey. I encourage the person to focus their attention on their mind's eye. With the aid of the medicine, the scenes are usually very clear but sometimes that is not the case. I ask them to let me know what's happening and what they see. If someone can't find an image that feels like their soul, that's okay; I instruct them to try to find a way of connecting with the soul to listen for some response. It's also okay if you lose the image temporarily.

I ask the participant to narrate any responses they receive back from the spirit world. I use concise and straightforward sentences because it's hard for journeyers to engage with complex language, due to the depth of the medicine's influence. I also do not want to give too much away to them, because I am not trying to add to the experience, only to get the journeyer to go deeper within their own psyche. The intelligence of the medicine and each individual's psyche are working together mystically. Still, I always have to be prepared for curveballs because the subconscious loves to play around. Being adept in navigating the terrain of the psyche takes a deep level of listening and experience on the part of the facilitator.

From the individual's responses, it quickly becomes clear how connected—or not—they are to their soul. Sometimes a person can't find any image of their soul at all. Or if it does appear, it will quickly fade away. Many people have no connection to their soul. I see this most commonly with individuals who are addicted to drugs like heroin and are receiving a more physical detoxification. For others, their soul may initially be unhappy or distrustful of them. Sometimes there is "cleanup work" to do—such as making peace with the soul and reconnecting before the soul is willing to answer the questions.

Let me show you another example of the soul kintsugi process, shared with the permission of the client involved.

Soul Retrieval

Stewart is a man in his late forties who was at times aloof when he came to me. I sensed he was an incredibly busy workaholic who carried some sadness. But he was disconnected from his emotions; it was too painful for him to acknowledge his feelings, which caused him to detach from his soul. When he was ready to engage in the process of soul retrieval, I sat beside him and began.

Keep in mind, when the journeyer is at this point, they are experiencing the peak of the iboga's effects. Forming complex sentences is not an option, yet they seem able to flow with the process.

ME: *Where do you live?*

JOURNEYER: *In a house.*

ME: *I want you to go to your front door and tell me when you're there.*

JOURNEYER: *Okay. I'm there.*

ME: *Go inside and find Stewart. Is he in the living room?*

JOURNEYER: *No.*

ME: *Is he in the kitchen?*

JOURNEYER: *No.*

ME: *What about in your bedroom?*

JOURNEYER: *Yeah, he's there.*

ME: *What is he doing?*

JOURNEYER: *He's lying on the bed.*

ME: *Say hi and let him know that you are happy to see him.*

[long pause]

ME: Ask him if he's okay with answering some questions.

[long pause]

ME: What's wrong?

JOURNEYER: I did see him, but he was arrested and taken off by the police.

[I think to myself, Wow, I've never encountered this before!]

ME: I guess we'll have to go down to the prison and visit him there. Let me know when you get there.

JOURNEYER: Okay, I am there.

ME: Great, I want you to go to the window and ask them if they have Stewart.

[he laughs]

ME: What did she say?

JOURNEYER: She said they have three Stewarts.

ME: Okay. Ask to see all three of them.

JOURNEYER: She's taking me to a room with a police lineup.

ME: Do you see Stewart in the lineup?

JOURNEYER: Yeah! He's the one on the right.

ME: Let's take him back home.

JOURNEYER: Okay, we are in the car together.

ME: Give Stewart a big hug. Let him know you're so happy to see him, and tell him you love him.

[long pause]

ME: Ask Stewart why he was arrested.

JOURNEYER: *He said it was mistaken identity.*

ME: *Where are you mistaken in your identity?*

[silence]

ME: *What's going on in there?*

JOURNEYER: *He's smoking a cigarette and drinking.*

ME: *Do you smoke?*

JOURNEYER: *No, but I used to.*

ME: *Ask him what's wrong.*

[seeing Stewart's soul smoking and drinking hinted that something was off]

JOURNEYER: *He says he's overwhelmed. It's too much to handle.*

ME: *Ask him what he needs from you.*

JOURNEYER: *He says, "a hug."*

ME: *Give him a hug.*

He gave himself a big heartfelt hug, reaching out and wrapping his arms around his chest on the bed. I could tell he was genuinely concerned for the well-being of his soul. His heart was opening to the authentic connection he and his soul were now experiencing. People often have profound emotional breakthroughs or tear up during this part of a journey. Imagine if it were you hugging your soul for the first time!

Stewart was a sensitive person with a robust and powerful mind. It seemed his soul had become imprisoned by that mind because he had ignored it, when all the soul really wanted was his acknowledgment and love. His soul went to great lengths to seek his attention, getting arrested for mistaken identity, drinking, and smoking—acting out just as a teenager might when needing attention.

After he'd offered love to his soul, that long-neglected soul still required digging and patience to be brought back into alignment. It needed deep presence, connection, and a hug—to be acknowledged and loved. Going back to the kintsugi metaphor, the "hug" was the magical glue necessary to bring his pieces back together, but at that stage, the glue was still wet. It needed time to set before it was ready to be painted with gold.

Stewart tells me that his life has changed since our journey. Before, he was not fully in charge of his own life. Now he gets up every day and greets to his soul in the mirror. He looks into his own eyes and connects beyond his superficial appearance to ensure that his soul feels loved. His continued practice of connecting to himself has illuminated his cracks with gold. When he looks me in the eye, I can see that his soul is ignited. A former serial entrepreneur, Stewart has turned to pursuing an artistic lifestyle. He feels more creative, more connected to himself, and more content with his life.

Once the soul connection has been forged, it's up to the individual to continue to cultivate a safe place for it to live; if it's neglected, it may go rogue again. And as with the art of kintsugi, once the glue sets, you also have to polish the edges. This is the daily work of integration. A person has to make space for their soul in everyday life, through practices like meditation, journaling, and ensuring that whatever they are is doing is aligned with their soul. Most important is to remind the soul you love it and always check in to see what it needs. In the practice of soul kintsugi, meeting the soul is like gathering the scattered pieces of oneself, acknowledging its presence, and understanding its needs and desires. The act of reconnecting is akin to applying the metaphorical glue, of the work of repair to bring one's soul back into harmony. Once the initial reconnection is made, offerings of love, compassion, and self-care represent the application of the metaphorical gold. This involves ongoing self-reflection, mindfulness practices, nurturing, and conscious choices aligned with the soul's needs and desires.

From Broken to Beautiful

As we have seen, soul kintsugi starts by observing the schism with one's soul. It means gently picking up the broken pieces to understand them and how they might fit together. Our self-knowledge and reconciliation of past events make up these pieces that slowly shape a bigger picture. This process requires deep presence and reflection. In Japanese kintsugi, the lacquer, which is known as *urushi*, and is made from tree sap, takes weeks to set. That is when we rest in stillness and focus on observing rather than doing. We may feel vulnerable or raw, like a newborn infant. This is the rebirth and the integration process.

Only through sitting with our feelings and focusing on the root causes of ongoing patterns and triggers can we truly get to a better place mentally. This is the work of inner alchemy, and it takes courage and discipline to face the uncomfortable spaces within. Most often, people don't want to feel anxiety or sadness. Some seek distraction by scrolling through Facebook, watching a movie, emotional eating, or drinking alcohol. The next time you have a distressing emotion, try sitting still and feeling it, even if you feel the urge to avoid it. Be curious about it. Ask what it wants. Usually these negative patterns are rooted in core safety issues that began in early childhood or were passed down from our ancestors. There is a myth that we must fix our flaws, but sometimes just being seen is all these parts need.

Anything negative we harbor creates pain within ourselves. Any time we act in hate toward another, we raise our blood pressure and trigger massive stress that lowers our immune system defenses and wreaks havoc within our bodies physically—not to mention the destabilization of inner peace, which can take time to restore.

But if we are able to slow down and become aware of the egoic aspect of ourselves, and to witness this part of ourselves rather than be consumed by it, insights gained become the glue that connects us back to our souls. This takes discipline and patience. But in every moment, we have a choice—the soul or the ego. Which do we choose to lead with? This is the ongoing practice of soul kintsugi. As we empower our souls to take the lead, we smooth the rough edges until doing so becomes second nature, and ego and soul become one.

How do you feed your soul? Do you engage with it every day? Are there frenetic times when you might fly through the day without pausing, being present, and looking to your soul? If you commit to a daily self-care or spiritual practice—such as yoga, nature walks, journaling, meditation, or regular healing of trauma through the alchemical process—you'll form a deeper relationship with your inner world.

This higher state of connection must be a deliberate lifestyle choice. In each passing moment, we can choose either to lean inward and compassionately evolve, nurture ourselves, and stay connected with our souls—or do what has been our societal norm: disassociate from our souls, self-soothe, and run away. Instead, when we become soul-centered we learn to trust our intuition and follow our hearts. Psychedelics and plant medicines can support us in taking the leap inward, as they can reveal our blind spots and open our eyes to new possibilities.

If we set a course of creativity and heart-inspired action, we will manifest our true desires for ourselves in this life. And when bumps in the road arise, we'll know this is simply another opportunity to practice soul kintsugi. To quote a popular saying often attributed to Stoic philosopher Marcus Aurelius, "Whatever stands in the way is the way." The path to healing, which ultimately leads to your highest joy, comes as a side effect of following your truth, the way of the artist. The artist recognizes that we always practice our art to develop our skills and evolve. Our healing happens naturally as we follow our artistic, creative path.

As you follow this path, not everything will work out perfectly. There will be places where we are stymied and blocked. This is where we pause, go inside ourselves, and ask questions. Let the answers come to you. I will equip you with some intuitive tools in chapter 9 to help you develop this skill for yourself. Be patient. Let go of your attachments and preconceived notions and try to understand the nature of your issue and address potential obstacles. Before moving ahead, wait until you've achieved clarity and received a signal and then ask for signs. This does not mean your visions for life achievements or successful will come overnight; it means you're true to yourself and your unique path and create a life that has meaning for you—which is what brings fulfillment and joy in the end. The act of seeding consciousness requires us to hold the dimensional complexity of both the ego and the soul simultaneously—in chapter 3 we learned how to listen to and identify these parts. Now, we're using acceptance and compassion as the gold to piece them together.

How can we practice soul kintsugi every day? This begins by listening closely to our thoughts, listening for the ego's voice, and consciously empowering the voice of the soul. Start a journal to record each of these voices. Can you learn to distinguish between the hungry ghosts of the ego and the surge of spark from your soul? On the next page I lay out some of the core beliefs associated with the voice of the ego—false beliefs that block your self-connection, creativity, power, and feelings of wholeness as well as reinforce destructive patterns in your life.

There are tools to help inform this process, like the Enneagram, which goes into depth on the shadow aspect of the ego, but my goal is not to get you caught up in some dogma or system of rules. I want you to feel these things and to know them by the practice of feeling them within yourself. When you get too reliant on personality tests or pre-set categories, you risk losing the magic of feeling the path within and its unexpected discoveries. While these types of tools can help you understand the bigger picture, they ultimately only provide a framework for a path that already exists deep inside you. The more you learn to see it, the less you need the tools.

. . . .

SEEDING CONSCIOUSNESS IN PRACTICE

Everyday Soul Kintsugi

For this exercise, reflect on the limiting beliefs below, and take note if and when they have come up for you. You may choose to write your thoughts in a notebook. After completing the exercise, ask yourself, how often is the ego chiming in, and how often are you letting your soul's voice lead?

The Egoic Voice

Sometimes your inner dialogue might be overwhelming. But by recognizing the soul and making soul-empowering choices, you can counter the voice of the ego. So which voice do you choose to believe? How do you feel when you engage with your soul?

"I don't belong."

> This kind of thought can manifest as "checking out" (disassociation) or isolation. It can also show up when comparing yourself to other people. No one should be compared to someone else. Our uniqueness is the signature and strength of the soul. Also, our perception of others through the lens of the ego tends to put them on a pedestal, and we can often inadvertently give our power away.

"I can never get what I want."

> When we put a carrot on a stick, it is always beyond our reach. Even the language we use, such as "I will get . . . " or "I'm going to . . . " puts our satisfaction in the future tense, which separates us from it.

"I deserve it."

> Life is a gift: nothing is owed to anyone, and there are no guarantees. When we feel entitled to something, we never truly enjoy it because we have no gratitude for the grace we've received, and do not appreciate its worth. This is about letting go of attachments to things and situations.

"I make things happen in life."

> When we exert force, we exhaust ourselves and can miss opportunities

for listening and allowing the universe to show up for us. A pattern of pushing can leave little room for joy or wonder. When we act from a place of fear, we often end up manifesting things that don't benefit us or that we did not really want in the first place. The salve for this wounding is around stepping into receptivity and allowing.

"I don't have enough time, money, or energy."

We will never be satisfied if we approach life from the perspective of scarcity. The lack comes from our feeling that what we have is not enough. For instance, a lack of energy may come from one's inability to relax and rest. Perhaps our anxiety won't allow our minds to switch off. These negative patterns are often rooted in core safety issues that began in early childhood. Being grateful for what we do have allows more to come our way and opens the space for grace.

"I don't deserve to be happy."

Sometimes we push things away—like love, success, and happiness—because we feel we are not worthy of them. Likewise, when feelings like these arise, we may also engage in self-destructive behavior. Worthiness goes far beyond who we are and what we think we have or don't have. Letting go of shame and guilt and bringing in forgiveness can help lighten the feelings of being deserving. The sun shines on every creature, the Earth holds them, and the water cleanses them. Every breath is a gift and an affirmation of our value.

"I'm anxious or afraid."

Fear is activated in the animal part of the brain, which is reactionary and tends to act hastily. Excitement can also create the same biological responses in the body, such as an increased heart rate, but is typically viewed as positive. Acknowledge where you feel the fear in our body. Comfort that part of yourself. Allow it to pass like a storm.

"I'm not enough."

When we feel inadequate, we often surrender our agency, seeking external approval rather than trusting our inner worth. Our essence is inherently whole and complete. Feeling small can lead us to shrink from opportunities and silence our voice. These feelings frequently stem from childhood experiences of bullying, abuse, or domination. Thus this sense of unworthiness is a self-enforced fiction that distorts the reality of who we are at our core essence.

"They're taking my power away."

The "us versus them" mentality is prevalent in political parties, politically oriented individuals, and activism movements. It manifests as a fight against the "bad guys" rather than seeing the "other" in ourselves. Here, I don't intend to overlook real injustices or their victims but rather to warn against conflict-based mindsets that create more victims. Over-identifying with such narratives can keep our souls in prison and prevent us from discovering and activating the infinite power within. It puts the responsibly on the other, rather than on our own reparative processes. Boundaries are paramount for a healthy psyche, so look for where there is agency to create them. That might mean expressing hurts or being firm, but if we are reliant on others' compliance, it further imprisons us through giving our control and power away.

The Soul Voice

When we are connected to the soul, the same experiences we reviewed above can yield different reactions. Let's take a look.

"Let me feel this."

Suffering exists to teach compassion. Compassion is the ability to access love even at the most difficult times or for the most seemingly undeserving recipients. We avoid feeling because, many times, it's painful. Humans are powerfully emotive beings; this is a blessing and a curse. We must learn to regulate ourselves by resisting the urge to react to external events. In the most difficult moment, can you pause to take a breath and drop deep into feeling? Accessing our emotional experience is the path to the soul. As Neale Donald Walsch, the author of *Conversations with God*, shares, "Feeling is the language of the soul. If you want to know what's true for you about something, look to how you're feeling about it." This gift of welcoming the full spectrum of our emotional experience is an act of love.

"I trust life."

We come to understand that we live in a friendly universe by feeling safe in the world and enjoying inner peace. We trust that the future holds positive potential. A degree of openness allows us to receive gifts from the universe. This does not mean there is no danger in the world; any danger that exists must be acknowledged. Yet beyond the ego and feelings of suffering, an overarching intelligence supports and animates all forms of life that we can connect to through our intuition.

"I'm grateful."

Understanding that life itself is a gift means feeling gratitude and appreciation for it, no matter what happens. Forgiveness, compassion, and sympathy toward yourself and others flow from having a humble or beginner's mindset. Cultivating gratitude even when you don't have it doesn't mean bypassing what is present in the moment, including feelings that need to be integrated. It means the practice of being grateful is part of how we generate feelings of love and keep our hearts open.

"Whatever is beneficial for me will be provided."

Have faith that all your needs will be supported, so long as they align with your path. Having to chase things or force them to happen usually means it's for the wrong reasons. You might even manifest that thing, but there is usually a cost—in the form of a karmic lesson. The web of life is infinitely abundant and cares for you. When you align to it, it's better attuned to what you communicate, and you don't waste your time unconsciously manifesting things that you clearly don't want. Both the ego and soul are informing it, whether you are aware of it or not.

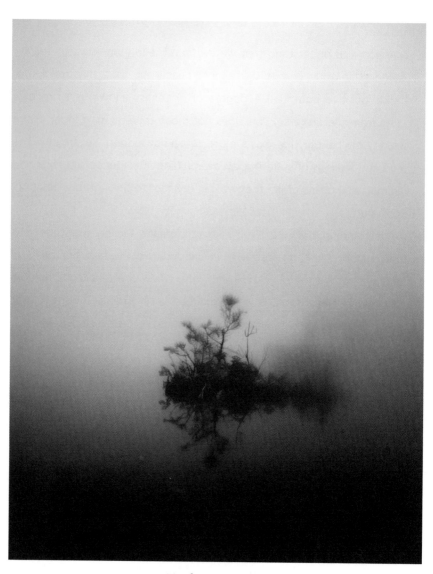

Teach Me to Forget

by Lela Amparo

5
Learning How to Die
Seeding Consciousness through Ego Death

When the ego dies, the soul awakens.

MAHATMA GANDHI

The process of initiation many times leads to a mystical experience resulting what is known as "ego death." Often these experiences inform our practice of soul kintsugi. Many of us fear death, the great unknown. Our society represses the dark aspects of nature. Jivanmukti, the founder of Siddhanta Yoga Academy and author of *Invoking Reality*, states, "Because we do not know life, we are scared of death. If we knew what life is, we would not differentiate life or death." But, often, for us to find peace and live in harmony with life we must metaphorically reenter the womb to reconnect to our inner wisdom. In essence, we must first die before we can truly live, diving into the depths of our suffering to access our power and recognize the truth of who we are. This is the purpose of initiation. Through use of psychedelics, plant medicines, and ancestral rituals that incorporate these psychoactive substances, we can learn how to die.

Poet Jessica Sevapreet Hesser imparted, "The death cycle will take you closer to your wild parts, the ancient ones, the parts that know death well. And they will tell you more about yourself than any book or master." This is because the "ego death" process is known to shift how people perceive themselves in relation to the world. Ego death speaks to the loss of self-identity or individuated consciousness. Carl Jung would refer to this state as the "psychic death."

Meanwhile, common throughout Taoist literature is the notion that enlightenment can be achieved only through the darkness, which connects to our origins: that is, nothingness. Experiences with psychedelics and plant medicines give us a taste of the feeling of ego dissolution, leading to a "nothingness," which is, in essence, a simulated death. This surrender to the dying process can feel scary but reminds us that the nature of life is always transient and impermanent and that both the good and bad in our lives play a role in the creative process that shapes every facet of us.

Everything we need to know about how to handle death, and the changes that come in rebirth, can be seen in the natural world. Observing the natural world teaches us how we, as humans, can tap into our creative power to become more adaptive to change. The sequoia tree is a great example of how we can turn death into opportunity. The seeds need the intense heat of the fire to germinate. The fire, in turn, loosens the soil to allow the seedling to grow solid roots and take in the carbon from the ashes of the burnt-down forest, providing rich nourishment for this massive tree to rise—like a phoenix rising from the ashes.

The story of the sequoia can also help us recontextualize why we may have experienced traumatic events. Can our own adversities, those times of pain or distress when we are forced to surrender our attachments to how we and the world "should" be, become the catalysts that bestow immunity and strength upon us? Trauma is like the fire that births the sequoia: when we know how to face and work with our pain, this awareness can allow us to grow stronger and evolve. What if instead of resisting or running from adversity, we catalyze it to harness the creative forces within? Combustion powers engines, and the Bwiti say the big bang set forth the beginning of creation in the cosmos. Embracing the flames and knowing how to walk with the element of fire allows you to clear the path for new seeds to germinate in our lives.

While our culture encourages us to numb or run from adversity, psychedelics and psychoactive plant medicines can turn up the heat of the fire, bringing everything to the surface to be purged, released, and cleared to create space for new life. Practicing ego death through the use of psychedelics or other transcendental catalysts matters because if we never experience ego death, we may continue to operate from our old trauma-based conditioning, never fully surrendering to the great mystery of life. Perpetually carrying the weight of the fears and tension our bodies cling to is like living in a house full of accumulated junk. As a result, we may live in a reactive state and feel stuck, seeing threats everywhere. We become trapped in small, overly guarded lives, hindering our ability to realize our full sovereign potential. In the words of Matshona Dhliwayo, Canadian author and philosopher, "A seed neither fears light nor darkness, but uses both to grow."

When you undergo a psychedelic experience, many people first have a disorienting sensation of losing control, which can cause fear or discomfort. Some people become nauseous. You might also sweat, shake, cry, or even laugh. These are signs of the ego being purged—which is part of the purification process of inner alchemy. And this is a process we are in collectively right now. Both humanity and the planet we inhabit are going through a deep cleansing process, a cleansing that is needed as we enter a new phase of creation. Like the blackened forest after a fire, we've entered a liminal space. In order to step into a place of balance with the natural world so that humanity can thrive, we must make important choices about aligning with the destructive ego or the creative soul. It might sometimes feel lonely or uncertain, living in what feels like a deconstructive void. But only when we learn how to die can we be reborn.

The Practice of Ego Death

I believe we get stuck and suffer from the malaise of disconnection because our society lacks metaphorical ways to practice "death." Using such practices would help us face and accept the suffering and sense of loss connected with change. Transience is the nature of all life. We must learn to move and transition through the twists and turns that are part of being alive and truly living. This is why many ancient initiations simulate death—ego death. Rituals around death and mystical experiences can help us shed the layers of old psychic conditioning, letting us evolve as individuals, develop resilience to change, and master the art of letting go.

One reason we are so afraid of death is that we believe time—and therefore life—is finite. For example, when I have guided people in using 5-MeO-DMT, the most common thing they say when they return is: "How long was I gone for?" In our culture we've been conditioned to obsess about time, when life and Creation are infinite, transcending time and space. Psychedelics and plant medicines teach us this. When we enter into these transpersonal states—particularly using a substance like 5-MeO-DMT, which works rapidly in dissolving the ego and switching off the default mode network—often we can understand and process information at light-speed, literally. Time can feel like eons passing in a blink, or it can stop completely. What does this say about our limited perception of time? Time is much more than hands on a clock or days in a calendar year. In fact, our experience of time is shaped by our state of consciousness. Time travels in cycles, stretching or constricting in descending and ascending spirals. The "days" get shorter in the winter and longer in the summer due to the Earth's position relative to the Sun—from this, we see that time is naturally cyclical and dynamic. The ancient Mayans understood this, and measured time with careful precision, according to the cycles of the universe.

When a person ingests the psychedelic medicine 5-MeO-DMT, often they enter into a non-dual state of being. Nonduality is the state of pure consciousness, where one experiences complete wholeness from a perspective beyond the limits of personal identity imposed by the ego. During such experiences, our consciousness merges at the speed of light into a higher vibrational and dimensional perception of time. Nonduality can also be described as the experience of unitive consciousness.

Deep in this non-dual state is the void, which is complete nothingness—a total blackout. I have witnessed the ego pop in during the experience and be completely disoriented. The journeyer might ask, "am I dead?" I quietly remind them they are ok and to let go. Some have the realization that we are all just specks of dust and that life—the degrees one has accumulated, and all the other material accomplishments—are ultimately insignificant. To the ego, this can feel like the end. All that drive, all that fight—for what? Again, this is a game the ego is playing, asking questions to maintain its status within this cosmic moment when the only thing to do is *just surrender*.

When I support somebody in this experience to help them to let go, I will remind them that surrender requires you to relax every inch of it your body—to breathe into the places of tension. Maybe your jaw is clinging on for dear life or your fist is tightly clenched. You can reassure yourself that it's okay. You are safe. If you feel tension or pressure, that's normal. It's like going through the birth canal; but it's only temporary. The tension will soften much faster if you breathe through it without judging the experience or trying to track what is happening. Use your breath to pull yourself out of the stress response. Inhale for ten seconds through your nose and breathe out for ten seconds through your nose. Keep cycling your breath in this way to regulate your nervous system. The breath is key!

The safety that the ego seeks in its attempts to control, or resist, is often based upon ancient programming. Undoubtedly our ancient ancestors had to respond instinctually to frequent physical threats; sometimes we need these survival instincts too. However, perpetually operating from this survivalist programming is an out-of-date response. "Role playing" death, using the concept of ego death, allows these survival patterns to be reprogrammed and fine-tuned in a safe, supported space, so they are not overly reactive, releasing a lot of the suffering we impose on ourselves. In essence, the practice of learning to die before you die creates space for you to live.

Part of the process of ego death is letting go of the old. Modern society has ignored the importance of honoring death and proper grieving. Many of us are carrying around heaps of grief, fear, and anger. The load may feel so unbearable that some part of us can't imagine facing this beast inside. But with practice, we can teach our bodies to express rather than repress our emotions. Experiencing trapped emotions in altered states is a great opportunity to learn to recognize and work them out.

Surrender. What does that mean? In medicine work, it means to resist the urge to track your experience or make it mean anything while it's happening; to be in the moment, listen, feel, and receive. There will be plenty of time to unpack it later. The grasping ego fears it will forget some important detail, but the lesson here is that we must choose to trust. We will always remember what we need to remember. Excessive clinging during a journey can often prevent another, more expansive wave of experience or deeper revelations from coming through.

As you drop into this place of receptivity, the different parts of yourself will begin to speak, one by one. Your legs might start shaking. Let them shake. This is how trauma is released from the body. Don't open your eyes. Stay inward. Keep allowing. If you feel sick, don't worry; keep letting go. You may throw up, but you will feel lighter and more open if you do. We can trust these time-tested tools' intelligence as they work through our bodies. For now, there's no need to reflect on what you're releasing from deep within. Keep surrendering.

And once you have learned how to die—by which I mean *let go* of the painful emotions and limiting, fear-based egoic patterns that have come to define you—you will often emerge feeling waves of bliss and peace in your body, and a restored sense of trust in the greater design of life. If you reach this point, congratulate yourself; you fully surrendered! It is no easy feat.

It is normal for people to come to this work with a great deal of fear. This is because the ego always wants control, believing that controlling our environment creates "safety." Individuals will often ask about the dosage and attach concerns about taking more. As much as information might give you peace of mind, the real secret is to breathe and allow. We can ease into the work bit by bit.

Once someone has a mystical experience, it gives them a new understanding of who they are, and a glimpse of something other than the suffering they so greatly wanted to be free from. But when the ego comes back online, it often tries to pick everything apart. Was that real? What did it actually mean? Sometimes the experience is rejected or forgotten by the conscious mind—and this is when the work really begins. Going forward, we must remember that learning how to die means learning to trust once again in the universal principles of life.

What I have learned the most through my work is that ego death is a beautiful thing, and typically those who dip their toe in the great mystery weep tears of gratitude and recount it as one of the most important experiences of their lives. Our fear of death is rooted in our own resistance to it and the suffering that this resistance creates inside us. As psychedelic research pioneer Bill Richards told his patients, "If you experience the sensation of dying, melting, dissolving, exploding, going crazy, etc., go ahead. Experience the experience."

This simulated "death," ego death, helps us to die and be reborn every day. Feeling and moving through difficulties in a psychedelic journey builds resilience. In life, we will experience pleasure and suffering, but when we lean only into pleasure and do whatever we can to avoid suffering, we halt the natural creative process. This causes us to accumulate unmetabolized, challenging emotions in our bodies, such as fear and shame.

Rather than reacting, the experience of facing ourselves and our fears when under the influence of the medicine teaches us not to react to outside stimuli. This in turn allows us to stay open, receptive, and curious. As we maintain this presence, we are able to move through situations more quickly. And over time, we learn how to direct energies in more constructive ways. As the German poet Johann Wolfgang von Goethe stated, "Death is Nature's expert advice to get plenty of Life." When we learn to die, we create space to live more fully.

Initiation by Darkness

Ego death is a central theme and process in many ancient traditions, with the act of plunging someone into darkness being used as a literal simulation of death and dying. These rites also mirror what can be experienced in a psychedelic journey. For example, the pyramids of Egypt were not only burial chambers for kings but also places where these initiatory rites took place during pre-dynastic times. Ancient civilizations expert Freddy Silva backs up the claim that the sarcophagi—the stone funeral receptacles for a corpse or mummy—inside of the King's Chamber of the Great Pyramid were used for special initiatory rites that created a mystical, out-of-body experience, perhaps similar to a high-dose psychedelic journey with 5-MeO-DMT or psychoactive plants. One rite in Kemetic (ancient Egyptian) initiations involved being closed inside a sarcophagus for three days. It is believed that the adept, while sealed inside the sarcophagus, experienced a death and rebirth, resulting in a mystical awakening. This experience planted a seed that grew within from a place of being reborn, helping the initiate remember their true essence, which takes seat in the heart.

The initiation by darkness described in Kemetic scriptures resembles some techniques found in other traditions. The Taoist teacher Mantak Chia, for example, holds meditation sessions in complete darkness. Students of tantra meditate in dark caves, following the teachings of Tantric Buddhist teacher Padmasambhava. These extend to thirty- or forty-day "dark retreats" designed to give participants an experience of *bardo*—that liminal space between life and death As previously described, an even more extreme example is the Kogi mamos, who are chosen through divination to begin an initiation involving at least nine years of living in a dark cave. This is because it is believed that being enveloped in darkness is how we return to a sense of primordial wholeness—returning to the womb of the mother, the great void. In the darkness, all we can do is listen, receive, and allow. When we eliminate artificial light, we start to see with our interior light.

So what is actually happening when we spend extended periods in darkness? According to Hood's Mysticism Scale, transcendent consciousness, or the mystical experience, is typically ineffable, timeless, spaceless, sacred, noetic in quality, real, and ultimately revelatory. Some methods for accessing these states include ingesting tryptamine-containing substances such as psilocybin mushrooms, 5-MeO-DMT, and ayahuasca. But what few know is that these psychoactive tryptamines are also endogenously produced, and breathwork, meditation, initiatic ritual, or extended periods in absolute darkness can equally help us access these "naturally" altered states.

In his book *Darkness Technology*, Mantak Chia explores the role of tryptamine synthesis in the body and brain. According to Chia, prolonged exposure to darkness builds up an excess supply of melatonin in the brain until it reaches a tipping point at which the pineal gland converts melatonin into the "spirit molecules" DMT and 5-MeO-DMT, along with pinoline and serotonin. These endogenous psychoactive molecules interact with neurotransmitters, inducing a unitive experience that echoes the Sufi poet Rumi's enumerations on unitive consciousness: "You are not a drop in the ocean. You are the entire ocean in a drop."

As a medicine woman, I have worked with individuals for nearly a decade using the powerful psychedelic 5-MeO-DMT. Typically smoked, the experience of 5-MeO-DMT invokes an extremely direct, intense flood of coherence in the brain resulting in feelings of connection and compassion. In my explorations of different states of consciousness, I became curious about how 5-MeO-DMT could produce a feeling to match the embodied sense of oneness that results from gamma wave brain states, which can also be induced through holotropic breathwork, sound healing, flotation tank therapy, or a lifelong meditation practice. Gamma wave brain states, between 25 and 140 Hz, are associated with feelings of a unitive state of consciousness, oneness, and connection—the highest expressions of coherence in the brain. Buddhist traditions may refer to degrees of these states as samadhi, nirvana, satori, or enlightenment—all of which speak to the state in which we feel completely whole and at peace and in which the ego is offline.

One could even go so far as to say that gamma is the opposite of the state of addiction, which is characterized by endless consumption or seeking to find wholeness, oneness, and connection. Chances are you've felt gamma yourself already; temporary spikes in gamma occur when we see a beautiful scene in nature, like a sunset, or we see someone we find beautiful, perhaps a baby or a person we love.

I also find it quite symbolic and metaphorical that the *Incilius alvarius* toad hibernates under the desert floor, *in total darkness*, for nine months of the year—the same length of time a human baby spends in the womb. Interestingly, the word *alva* in Latin means "of the womb," and in numerology, the number nine represents the end of a cycle. While underground, the toads enter a state of monk-like meditation. Drawing upon ancient practices along with these cycles of death and rebirth, one could hypothesize that a form of alchemy is taking place when, as a result of this exposure to darkness, the Sonoran Desert toad generates its essence, the bufotoxin, with gamma-inducing 5-MeO-DMT.

To test the hypothesis that 5-MeO-DMT induces gamma wave states within the brain, I collaborated with UCLA Professor Dario Nardi, Ph.D., who specializes in neuroscience research, to perform EEG brain scans on recipients of 5-MeO-DMT. EEG readings indicated increases in gamma brain waves while recipients were under the influence of 5-MeO-DMT. The brain was saturated in gamma brain waves, and there were spikes in the high gamma bandwidth in the brain. Studies conducted by the University of Wisconsin–Madison show that Zen Buddhist monks with a lifelong practice have significantly high gamma waves while meditating. Monks or meditators with a practice developed over decades have referred to gamma brain states as experience of grace or being blessed. The states associated with high gamma wave oscillations are viewed in some traditions as the utmost state of enlightenment, in essence the alchemist's philosopher's stone.

A gamma state benefits the brain by increasing memory recall, focus, perception, and the ability to process vast amounts of information, as well as bringing about a positive, grateful mood and sense of peace. On rare occasions, gamma activity triggers a constellation of neurons that work synergistically to create new neural network pathways and overall harmonization in the brain. Gamma creates high levels of coherence in the brain, which can cause bursts of insight, or "aha" moments. Modern mystics and biohackers alike use psychedelics and these ancient practices to boost gamma and access the most intense flow states.

Reports of "reactivations" of the gamma wave state after using 5-MeO-DMT are also commonplace. Many individuals who work with 5-MeO-DMT describe a further ease in accessing gamma wave states during meditation, acupuncture, or floatation tank therapy. I believe 5-MeO-DMT creates a bridge or pathway to this state of consciousness, making it more readily accessible after the experience. Might gamma brain waves be the bridge of the reclamation of the soul and the indicator of a transcendence or mystical rebirth?

The Path to Transcendence

In the paper, "The Varieties of Self-Transcendent Experience," by Johns Hopkins University professor and researcher David Yaden, researchers assert that the states of ego death, mystical experience, awe, and flow—with given variability in the intensity of perceived unity—encompass degrees of Self-Transcendent Experiences (STE).

We can see that high gamma wave oscillations on EEG readings are associated with these self-transcendent states. But what is actually happening to us when we experience them? Perhaps the mystics may have the answer. The Buddhist and Vedic traditions associate the states of ego death with a movement of life force energy, known as prana or kundalini. Vasant Lad, an Ayurvedic doctor whom many regard as the godfather of Ayurveda, describes kundalini as a neuroelectrical energy that is the gateway to the inner journey. In my lineage of Bwiti Fang, we call this *mboumba eyano*, which translates to the energy of the soul, or what might be understood as quintessence. It is the part of ourselves that is most important to stay connected to, as we will be lost without it. In initiation we learn what our *mboumba eyano* represents mystically. One thing is clear, we must engage with our kundalini to discover what it is for ourselves. When flowing freely, kundalini is the source of our creativity, connecting us to the web of life and beyond. When we live from our egoic template, kundalini becomes trapped, stagnant, or blocked, and it can lead to illness or malaise. During psychedelic initiation and/or ego death, kundalini is freed to move throughout the chakras, which facilitates a transcendent experience.

Kundalini, symbolically represented by the serpent, two to be exact, starts out coiled at the base of the spine, at the root chakra. When the chakras are open, kundalini is free to travel up the spine and through all the chakras. In Egyptian cosmology, kundalini energy is referred to as the tongue of Thoth, or P'tah (an aspect of Thoth), because the tongue utters the first sound, beginning the creative process and leading to the manifestation of wisdom in the initiate. And so, as kundalini uncoils and rises through your spine, you are beginning to access the wisdom of Thoth; that is, the wisdom that humans are powerful, multidimensional beings.

The term *animism* is linked to the belief that all things are alive. It is true all atoms vibrate and all things, even if they appear solid, are in a state of change and movement, some just vibrating faster than others. You can think of kundalini as the electricity, or charge, that animates all life. As Jana Dixon, spiritual teacher and author of *Biology of Kundalini*, advises us: "Consider that the fire that Prometheus stole from the Gods was actually Kundalini fire, and he gave it to the people so they could become Gods." I think of kundalini as the rocket fuel that allows our souls to travel beyond the physical world. But more on that later. Kundalini is the power behind the magic and the mystery; it is what powers the web of life. The spark within drives you to action, either creating abundance and beauty on Earth, or burning out and living an unfulfilling life in which you are giving away your power or seeking thrill.

Now that I've witnessed medicine journeys over the last decade, I've come to believe that the psychedelic journey activates the movement of kundalini through the chakra system. The alkaloids in psychoactive plants and substances open up the chakras by stimulating specific neurotransmitters that create coherence patterns in the brain, allowing for a range of experiences that crescendo at ego dissolution. As the brain comes into coherence, the ego goes through stages of dissolution, and kundalini rises up the chakra system as if ascending floors in elevator. In my experiences of bearing witness to this process—particularly with 5-MeO-DMT—I frequently observe the energetic current of kundalini progressing through a person, apparently clearing blockages in the body by activating shaking and other forms of purging as it comes through the body's energetic centers as described in more detail below. In Dr. Stanislav Grof's groundbreaking research in holotropic breathwork, spiritual emergence and transpersonal psychology references the kriyas in Vedic yoga tradition in reference to kundalini awakening.

> The most striking among these are powerful sensations of heat and energy streaming up the spine, associated with tremors, spasms, violent shaking, and complex twisting movements. Quite common also is involuntary laughing or crying, chanting of mantras or songs, talking in tongues, emitting of vocal noises and animal sounds, and assuming spontaneous yogic gestures (mudras) and postures (asanas).

Having studied mystical teachings like *The Tibetan Book of the Dead*, I believe this process may be the same or similar to what one experiences at the moment of birth or death. Psychedelic journeying returns us to the state in which we are born, when kundalini is free flowing. When we incarnate, the archetypal energies transmitted throughout the universe weave themselves into the fractals of light that come together to form our souls—as we will see in the next chapter. These archetypes are expressed in your chakra system and will determine your dharma to some degree, personality traits, and path in this lifetime. As such, the seven main chakras within us reflect our connection to the entire solar system.

As we integrate with the trauma of life on Earth in a flesh suit, painful experiences in our upbringing, to which none of us is immune, create blocks in the chakra system. Pain, grief, and fear accumulate in these energy centers, and unless we know how to work with these emotions and release them, they remain stuck in the body, blocking the flow within the kundalini channel. Think of these blockages like the Drano commercial, where you can visually see the clog of debris in the clear pipe. This keeps us stuck in our egoic patterns, as informed by our trauma, and can prevent access to transcendent states of consciousness. Now, instead of living as the divinely inspired, creative being that is our primordial state, our energy becomes heavy and dense like lead. It is the experience of ego death or dissolution that allows kundalini to flow freely again.

Chakras

To understand this better, let's take a closer look at the chakra system as it correlates to what is experienced during a psychedelic journey. You have seven main chakras located along your spinal column, spaced from the base of your spine to the crown of your head. The chakras are each associated with a color and are ruled over by a specific planet, displaying the nature and characteristics of that celestial body.

The journey through the energy centers begins at the base of your spine, in the root chakra. The root chakra is associated with the color red and is represented by the planets Mars and Saturn. It is what grounds you to the Earth, and its energy is symbolically masculine. The root chakra relates to themes of material safety: our jobs, our homes, and our relationships with our bodies. When the root chakra is grounded and open, we act from a place of deep security, knowing that we have the right to be here and that we have deep support from the Earth.

The sacral chakra, located in our sacrum, is a bright orange color and represents our sexuality. It is the emotional body and is ruled by Pluto and Jupiter. This chakra is on the plane of the plant kingdom, where all trees and plants originate. It's associated with the archetype of the mother, and it carries the essence of nurturing and creative energy.

Usually these two lowest chakras, the root and sacral chakras, are where we find the highest density of trauma, often related to survival fears stemming from our childhoods and any ancestral trauma that has been passed down to us through our DNA. In the West, we exist in a state of manufactured scarcity, and we are not taught how to release emotions; it makes sense that this creates blockages in the lower chakras. As these chakras open, any trauma we hold here rises up to the surface like an inflatable beach ball submerged underwater. This part of the process can result in the shaking, purging, emotional flashbacks, and visions of traumatic events that people often experience at the onset of a psychedelic journey. But this purging is necessary if kundalini is to be freed to move from the denser chakras up to the subtle chakras.

Next comes the third chakra, located in the solar plexus, which burns a bright golden yellow. Governed by the Sun and Mars, the third chakra rules the life force found in all living creatures. It holds our inner child, will, and self-expression—as such, it is also the realm of the healthy ego. The highest expression of the solar plexus is our self-realization, which can liberate us from suffering and powerlessness. Kundalini flowing freely here allows the ego to dissolve as it moves toward the heart. At this stage, individuals can still feel blocked from surrendering to the experience, because this is when we say *sayonara* to the ego as it begins its dissolution.

At this stage, people often notice a palpable shift in energy or emotion. Typically this is where one starts to feel more open or expansive—a sense of arriving at a familiar and safe place. The fourth or heart chakra, located in the center of the chest is ruled by Venus and the Moon and is associated with a bright green color. It is where we experience gratitude and connection, which binds us emotionally to all other living beings. When kundalini reaches your heart, you've gone from caterpillar to butterfly; this is where the spiritual path, the path of the mystic, begins. We are no longer in the 3-D realm of the lower chakras. This is the gateway to the higher astral dimensions.

Beyond the heart, the fifth or throat chakra emanates a bright shade of turquoise or blue. This chakra, a bridge between the inner and outer worlds, is ruled by Mercury. The energy of the throat chakra reflects our inner reality, and the fact that we must speak our truth to manifest what we want to see reflected in the outer world. Staying silent or taking actions that are out of alignment with our intentions causes blockages here. When this happens, we cannot materialize what we desire. We may also manifest things that do not serve us. When kundalini moves freely here, it brings to mind the ancient spell of manifestation, "abracadabra," which means "I create as I speak."

Once the two kundalini serpents hit the sixth chakra, referred to as the third eye, located in the middle of the forehead, we discover the deep purple hue of the psychic realms. This sixth chakra is the logos of the universe, where our souls leave their bodies behind and travel the celestial realms. In this place ruled by Jupiter and Neptune, we delve into our past lives to meet with our ancestors or the ascended beings working with us. The third eye chakra sits directly above the pineal gland, the *epiphysis cerebri*, found in most vertebrates' brains. This endocrine gland is commonly understood to regulate our sleep and dream cycles and is also connected to our intuition, or sixth sense, from which our dreams emanate.

Finally, the seventh, or crown, chakra is where we experience unification and complete transcendence. It is where we connect to the limitless Source of divine energy ruled by Uranus. Once kundalini has reached this chakra and we have attained this level of awareness, we no longer see form, and we lose our sense of time. One second in the crown chakra can feel like a million years. Many people experience this realm simply as bright light and feel an overwhelming sense of complete awe and of being bathed in pure, unconditional love.

As we travel higher up the chakras, kundalini becomes less dense. It leaves behind form or matter, and moves into formlessness, or Spirit. And as we ascend, we access more complex meta-intelligence systems. I call them galactic ashrams; they are schools where our souls go to learn. This is where we can access psychic abilities and other superhuman powers. Paramahansa Yogananda spoke of these realms as "astral heavens."

This is what I experienced my first time taking DMT. When I entered this realm, I found myself in the center of a golden circular court surrounded by Krishna, Buddha, the *neteru*, Ganesha, Lakshmi, and maybe a hundred more deities, all looking down at me. Others talk about being visited by alien-like creatures or divine angelic beings. I believe these are not simply visions or hallucinations but can carry many different levels of significance. My experience as both initiate and guide, as well as Kemet teachings, provide evidence that when our kundalini rises to these higher chakras, our souls have left our bodies and we are traveling in purely immaterial dimensions. This could be why so many of us see the same entities on our psychedelic journeys; perhaps we are leaving third-dimensional reality and visiting other dimensional planes that are accessible to us all. And here, we discover that death is not the end, only the beginning.

Death and Transcendence

Transcendence, according to many perspectives, is achieved by facing and understanding our pain—something that much of humanity, in an effort to evade discomfort, invests a great deal of resources and energy in avoiding. Intriguingly, key researchers in the field of quantum mechanics, such as Sir Roger Penrose and Dr. Stuart Hammeroff, propose that the journey to consciousness is mediated through cytoskeleton microtubules. These tiny structures form networks in the brain, acting as electrochemical transistors that facilitate consciousness. This could start to explain the travels beyond the physical realms and what might be keeping some of us from reaching them.

Hammeroff and Penrose, through their Orch-OR theory, suggest that these microtubules or their generating activities serve as quantum gateways to higher intelligence that goes beyond our basic brain matter. I sense that delving into the intersection of pain, consciousness, and addiction could enable discoveries that lead to great evolution in an area that has been a thorn in humanity's side for many generations. Currently researchers are discovering drugs that target these specific ion channels and offer great promise as treatments for addiction. Addiction, although complex and multifaceted, is often a sign that someone is seeking outside stimuli to cope with suffering or discomfort. Addictions or the traumas from which they stem may disrupt critical pathways, specifically ion channels, involved in facilitating consciousness.

Although these pathways are complex and not yet fully understood, they perform roles that include mediating pain. Consequently, if we address what lies at the root of addiction, reactive behaviors, and fear, we could potentially open the door to consciousness via this quantum gateway, which can result in unexpected benefits and growth as we embrace the concept of ego death as discussed in this chapter.

The grasshopper mouse serves as an intriguing metaphor in this exploration. This wild, ferocious creature is more akin to a wolf than a typical mouse: it howls to claim it territory and actively hunts dangerous predators such as scorpions and snakes, thus overturning its position in the food chain. This desert-dwelling species has evolved to become immune to the venom of the highly poisonous Arizona bark scorpion. Researchers at Michigan State University discovered that this adaptation involves a protein that inhibits the effects of the scorpion's sting by acting on the Nav 1.8 ion channel. Further studies at the University of Indiana revealed that a peptide, produced by the mouse in response to the venom, acts as an analgesic, blocking subsequent pain. The pain-blocking protein functions by recognizing the venom, which triggers a gating mechanism. At some point, overcoming the instinctual urges that most mice succumb to such as fleeing and hiding, this species essentially developed super-mouse capacities—most likely out of necessity, to survive in the harsh desert.

Like the grasshopper mouse, we, too, might evolve our responses to negative stimuli by examining and understanding our pain and discomfort. This could help us transcend our reactive behaviors and subconscious programming to gain access to a greater quantum consciousness, allowing for us to evolve and thrive as a species. This transformative process might even deepen our understanding of our interconnectedness with the universe and help us discover novel approaches to dealing with suffering, trauma, and building resilience. There is always a gift that comes from leaning into the shadow.

As Greek poet, novelist, and folklorist Dinos Christianopoulos said, "They tried to bury us. They didn't know we were seeds." When we face our deepest fears or adversaries, they become the compost that fertilizes new growth. In essence, learning how to die is an essential aspect of seeding our consciousness. Our fear of death often keeps us in unconscious patterns, avoiding things or clinging on rather than embracing change. Each time we remember to surrender, we plant that seed that opens the doorway for greater freedom. Through the practice of ego death, the blocked channels in the chakra system can open. What is preventing the universal life force energy from flowing through an individual can be decomposed for new life to begin to trickle through.

Keep in mind that these concepts like chakras or kundalini are helpful because they serve as a raft in the vast sea of consciousness. Buddha spoke, however, of how we only need the raft (or teachings) until we don't need the raft anymore. It's easy to get overly fixated on concepts and lose the point of the journey itself. The journey is about letting go of what you know and setting off into the unknown. I must warn you that when we are not ready or properly prepared for ego death, we can be spun sideways and tossed against the rocks. This is why many initiations happen in a sequential process. Even in some Buddhist traditions, many years of developing the root chakra through meditation are required before accessing more advanced tools. The serpent path of awakening kundalini starts from the root chakra as a slow and staged process, for good reason, because these latent energies that live inside us are incredibly powerful and when activated can bring chaos if not done with care. Unfortunately, the lightning path, a top-down approach starting at the crown chakra and moving quickly like a flash of electric voltage from the sky, is the main approach taken with psychedelics in Western culture. This can be very dangerous because of the level of trauma we collectively hold. When this energy gets activated, these traumas that live in our bodies rise up to be addressed. If too much comes up at once, it can be overwhelming or even retraumatizing. This is where the tools of inner alchemy, soul kintsugi, tuning in, and seeding consciousness act as a form of grounding, directing the energy to prevent it from expressing itself in harmful or disruptive ways.

The mystical experience and ego death hold the keys to one's truth but must be treated with the utmost respect, as it can be extreme or cause harm if not done properly. Working with a traditional practitioner or experienced facilitator is one way to ensure one is supported, prepared, and able to integrate the experience. In a study, "The Epidemiology of 5-methoxy-N, N-dimethyltryptamine (5-MeO-DMT) Use: Benefits, Consequences, Patterns of Use, Subjective Effects, and Reasons" in the 2018 *Journal of Psychopharmacology*, my partner, Joseph Barsuglia, and a team of researchers made a profound discovery regarding set and setting of 5-MeO-DMT, which ranks second highest in potent psychedelic experiences after ibogaine, or iboga.

The occurence of a complete mystical experience (based on the

Mystical Experiences Questionnaire (MEQ)*) among the group who were part of a ceremonial administration with a facilitator was thirty-three percent higher than those who experienced the non-ceremonial use of the same form of synthetic 5-MeO-DMT. The staggering increase in instances of mystical experiences speaks to the value of the ceremonial container that involves ritual, preparation, integration, and a facilitator capable of supporting one in navigating the terrain through ego death. Careful consideration must be taken in embarking into this territory. My hope is this knowledge will help guide that decision making process and remind others to take it slowly and mindfully on their path of activating theses powerful spiritual energies and embarking on mystical experiences.

As recording artist Seal sang, "We're never gonna survive unless we get a little crazy." Joseph is a mad scientist, and I mean that he brilliantly directs his out-of-the-box creativity to look at mystically-driven healing and its potential application on a societal level. Through the analysis of a text corpus of 569 experiential reports of 5-MeO-DMT, uploaded into AI GPT 4, AI expert and Nous Research founder Karan Malhotra posed a question based on the data set of these accounts: how can these encounters help humanity? The five distinct answers, taken from these compiled accounts, paint a picture of the potential benefits of self-transcendent experiences with psychedelics and plant medicines. The AI model said that 5-MeO-DMT has the potential to help humanity in several ways:

- fostering a sense of unity and interconnectedness
- emotional healing and personal growth
- encouraging spiritual exploration
- promoting a sense of gratitude, love, and compassion
- inspiring environmental stewardship

---

*The Mystical Experience Questionnaire is a psychometric scale designed to measure and quantify mystical experiences. It is based on the work of Walter Stace, a philosopher who studied mysticism and developed a common core model of mystical experiences that transcends specific religious or cultural contexts.

Within these insights lies a beacon of hope—a glimpse into a future where humanity embraces the profound lessons whispered by the molecules of creation. Through understanding and integration, the wisdom gleaned from these journeys may serve as a guidepost, illuminating the path toward a more connected, compassionate, and sustainable world.

We may not be able to experience an ego death through reading these pages, but meditating on death can help one to surrender and let go of fears about the finite nature of life. To close this chapter, let's embark on a journey into the inner world together, connecting to our deepest fears and "dying" to them so we can be reborn.

Some parts or even all of this meditation might be difficult for you. If you are vulnerable, it may not be the right time to try it. Remember, you can stop at any moment and open your eyes if you become overwhelmed. If you feel some discomfort, you can also welcome it and let it pass through, if you feel safe to do so.

· · · · · · · · · · · · · · ·

SEEDING CONSCIOUSNESS IN PRACTICE

Reflecting on Your Life after Death

To begin, find a comfortable position, sitting or lying down. If you tend to get cold, maybe place a blanket over your legs. First, take a moment to experience what it feels like to be alive. Take a deep breath in and let it out. Observe the sensations in your body—your nose hairs vibrating with the warm air from your lungs as you exhale, the rhythm of your heart beating, the feeling of your breath.

Now close your eyes and imagine you are looking out a window. Outside, it is spring, and you see green trees and flowers. You hear the rainfall as it feeds the soil. Then you blink, and it's summer. The Sun is shining, and the long days are filled with birds singing. Next, the leaves change color to autumn hues, painting a feeling of warmth. Then, slowly, the leaves turn brown, dry out, and fall from the trees. The landscape becomes stark, and snow begins to fall. Nature reminds us of the impermanence of things and the cycles of life. It never forgets its design, which is to die and be reborn over and over.

Now, see yourself as part of nature. Within you is this intelligent design that knows how to grow from a baby to puberty to an adult. Witness yourself getting old. You look down at your hands, and the skin gets dry and papery. You see age spots appear where there were none before. You are beginning to die. As your life force dissipates, you feel every muscle completely let go in your body. You feel your breath leaving your body and merging back into the atmosphere. Now you have left your body but are watching it from above. Time passes, and you notice signs of bloating and decay as your body begins its decomposition process.

Finally, see yourself as a pile of bones resting peacefully. But then you encounter a great light, and you walk toward it, the brightness almost blinding you. As you walk into the light fully, you enter a hallway. With each step, you are filled with the memories of your life, what you learned, and those you loved. Which memories and what lessons stand out to you? As you walk to the end of the hallway, you are greeted by others—guides and ancestors. They celebrate your arrival and embrace you with loving hugs. Maybe one of them has a message for you. Do you have something to say in answer? Take a moment to listen and receive. After you have received the messages, thank your guides and ancestors for coming to see you.

Now that you have visited the other side of death, begin to travel back to your body. Start to feel your consciousness return with your breath, as the life force energy fills your beating heart and circulates throughout your body, and imagine all the life essence of your being returning, revitalizing you as you return to your present age. Feel your feet on the ground beginning to awaken your body. And when you're ready, slowly open your eyes and let them adjust to the light in the room.

Was there anything that came up for you in that exercise? What do you notice about yourself after coming out of the experience? When you think about the idea of dying, does anything about it feel any different for you?

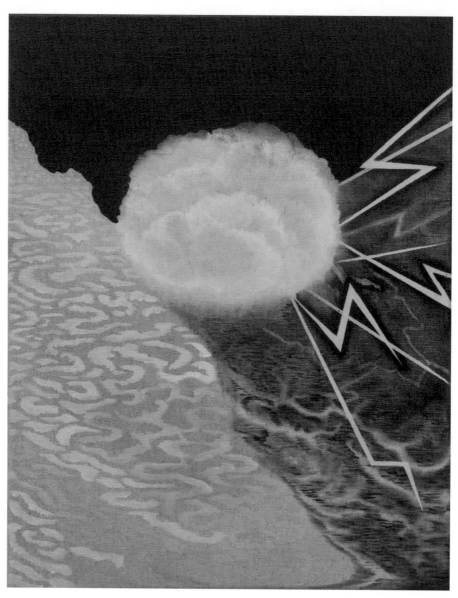

Resilience

by Katy Lynton

6

The Universe and the Innerverse

Exploring the Cosmos Within

Each human is a point of orientation through which the Universe experiences itself.

ADYASHANTI

Not until we have experienced ego death do we get to fully explore our innerverse—that inner world that is inextricably bound up with all that is. As with taking an adventure into the wilderness, we are limited to what things we can carry, and your journey to cross through the Bardo does not allow you to carry anything along. As mentioned in the introduction, when we traverse the innerverse—diving into the caves of our psyche to alchemize our densest material into gold—we perform a cosmic act of healing for the world. By freeing ourselves from the constraints of ego, we gain the ability to journey through this inner cosmos. This journey grants us a deeper understanding of and trust in life, illuminating our place within something far greater than ourselves.

As a child, I grew up close to the local library, where I spent most of my time reading books on folk craft and herbalism when I wasn't sewing, crafting, beading, weaving, or concocting. In my twenties I began my work in the wellness space, both studying and teaching aromatherapy, holistic healing, and shiatsu massage, which led me to the ancient knowledge systems that supported me as I sought answers to my deepest existential questions and healing. In my thirties I studied tarot, Human Design, Cha Dao—the ancient Chinese ritual of ceremonial tea rooted in Daoism—and alchemy. I was a student of life's mysteries long before I became a medicine woman, and I remain a lifelong student. These knowledge systems and my mystical experiences via initiation and altered states showed me that the innerverse within me and the universe I moved through were one and the same.

Through the course of my alchemical studies and experiences traversing my own innerverse, I began to grasp the workings of the psyche and how the archetypal energies act out through us, both at a cosmic and personal level. I slowly integrated, in an embodied way, what the ancients described as the universal forces of nature, their impact on us, and felt a sense of how we can work with these forces for spiritual healing and transcendence.

The equation of understanding our identity and place in the world is indeed intricate and mysterious. To comprehend who we are, our significance, and what contributions we can make, we must first acquaint ourselves with the vast architecture of existence in which we are inherently embedded. This chapter highlights the primordial wisdom that permeates all ancient knowledge systems. I hope my gathered reflections will deepen your understanding of this web of life.

It's bewildering to me that this profound interconnectedness is not more widely embraced, but I understand the complexity of it may be overwhelming for the egoic mind. This is not a dogma, it's a relational framework that points to our nature. The architecture of the symbolic mind comes through contemplative interaction; many answers are like a paradox that holds a point and no point at the same time. It can be everything and nothing and something else in relation to what is relating. The querant's inquiry just helps one move on the map. That means my interpretation is not yours and vice versa, yet there are always common threads.

As Above, So Below

One of the most famous tenets in alchemy is the concept of "as above, so below." This sentence is found in the *Corpus Hermeticum*, a text attributed to Hermes Trismegistus, the possibly mythic, possibly even real, Greek successor to the Egyptian god of wisdom, Thoth. This phrase can be interpreted to mean that while the entire universe is within us, everything within us is also present in the whole universe. We are the cosmos, and the cosmos is us, a mystical hall of mirrors stretching into infinity. There is a correspondence between the dense and less dense realities, which are perhaps mirrors or reflections of one another—an idea referred to as the Law of Correspondence, written in the Emerald Tablets, which describes how everything in the spiritual realm corresponds to the material realm. This "law" dictates that the divine is not separate from nature and the physical plane; rather, they are one and the same.

Many years ago, when I started mystery school, I read the Emerald Tablets of Thoth, a book written by the Egyptian deity of wisdom about the forty-two sacred tablets, which are inscribed with the secrets of the universe and the tenants of alchemy. I was so enthralled and immersed that I could not put the book down. That night Thoth came to me in a dream. He handed me a thick, weathered emerald tablet to hold for safekeeping. From that time forward, these laws of alchemy have played a big role in my life.

Today, the truths uncovered by the alchemists of old have been proven by modern science. Astrophysicists have shown that carbon, nitrogen, oxygen, and all the fundamental ingredients of life make up the human body and the cosmos. Many times in my work with iboga, the theme of the creation story was shown, beginning with a big bang. Gaseous stars birthed the elements, and from the elements formed matter, which eventually evolved from plants to amoeba to dinosaurs and then humans. But the ancient alchemists believed there was even more to it. They believed in the *metaphysical* nature of the cosmos—meaning that the stars and the planets embodied different forms of archetypal intelligence that could be felt but were not always seen. To mystics, the universe was both physical and metaphysical, as was humankind; just as our bodies were comprised of the physical materials that made up the whole, so too were our psyches comprised of the metaphysical elements of the universe.

This is another way of thinking about the innerverse. This inner world is often revealed to us in egoless, altered states of consciousness, a representation of the metaphysical universe that lives within each human, which, in turn, mirrors the entire cosmos. Because we can't see the metaphysical, some have forgotten that it exists. We're all capable of traversing the innerverse, but modern society has suppressed and even denied this aspect of ourselves. Yet our spiritual faculties can always be resurrected. They are always there, waiting for us, in the brain's right hemisphere—the side that speaks to us in symbols, coincidences, and intuition. This is the seat of our creative power and our connection to the archetypal energies of the cosmos. I also believe that humanity's more recent fascination with the mystical arts, including psychedelics and plant medicines, is due to a deep yearning to reconnect to this for-gotten and often suppressed part of ourselves and our history. When we're stuck in the logical left-brain realm, there is no magic or mystery, and life quickly becomes formulaic and sterile. As mystical teacher and author Manly P. Hall stated, "When the human race learns to read the language of symbolism, a great veil will fall from the eyes of men."

As I continued my studies, I began to understand how these meta-physical forces operated and how to work with them to manifest what I wanted for my life, in alignment with the greater principles of the cos-mos. This meant first letting go of what I "wanted"—which I realized was what the ego wanted—and using my body and intuition as guides to *what the greater web of life was leading me to.* As I discussed in the last chapter, this is the opposite of seeking; instead, it means acting on ideas that travel to us from the intuitive and creative realm, ideas that must go through the alchemical process from the ephemeral into matter. With this new information, I began to consciously create my life to align with the universal laws of nature, working with the energies that exist within and without, above and below.

Another basic alchemical tenet is that everything is energy. The Law of Vibration, written in the Emerald Tablet, states that everything, including thought and emotion, is a manifestation of energy vibrating at various frequencies. The material or three-dimensional world, which we experience as the physical realm of existence, is made of molecules that vibrate slowly and consistently, which is why they appear solid. In his book *Egyptian Cosmology: The Animated Universe*, Moustafa Gadalla explains that the Egyptian ancients believed in more quintessential dimensions than we experience in the material world—an idea later proven by modern physics. In these dimensions, Gadalla writes, molecules vibrate much more quickly, making things less dense. These subtle energy realms, as some call them, make up the metaphysical or spirit world.

Our senses are typically only attuned to what is in the third dimension: things we can see, touch, taste, smell, and hear. But as inventor Nikola Tesla once said, "If you want to find the secrets of the universe, think in terms of energy, frequency, and vibration." When we are caught in materialistic thinking, we limit ourselves to the densest levels of consciousness. When we transcend the limits of the mind and travel beyond language to the realm of the symbolic or right brain, more complex forms of intelligence can reach us.

And yet we in the modern world have shunned and belittled the metaphysical and multidimensional aspects of reality. As a result, so many of us have forgotten our true nature, and this spiritual amnesia causes us, as a species, to suffer greatly. Rather than seeing the whole picture and understanding both the material and metaphysical nature of life, we have lives that lack gratification, and we never fully tap into the great support that's right there at all times, waiting for us to ask. Our denial of the spirit world and our metaphysical nature has put our planet near extinction, as we have become unable to see that our individual suffering is directly related to the suffering of our planet.

Sadly, the world is full of disembodied people living within the confines of their egos and minds. These traumatized souls have suffered greatly from the severed connection between the universe and the innerverse. As elder "uncle" Angaangaq Angakkorsuaq of the Kalaallit Nunaat Nation in Greenland says, "The greatest distance in the existence of Man is not from here to there, nor from there to here. Nay, the greatest distance in the existence of Man is from his mind to his heart. Unless he conquers that distance, he can never learn to soar like an eagle and realize his own immensity within."

Cosmically Connected

You can think of the relationship between the universe and the innerverse as a series of nonlinear, interlinked programs operating dynamically and within a defined order as part of a larger system. But before we explore how the universe and the innerverse are connected, it is important to understand the cosmic order that forms the basis of our solar system. Through my studies and in my medicine journeys, I have seen that within all the systems in our cosmos, there is an order. As Paul Brunton, a British author with an extensive background studying the Hindu and Esoteric knowledge systems, puts it, "There is an established order in the universe, scientific laws which govern all things, and no magician who seems to produce miracles has been permitted under special dispensation to violate that order or to flout those principles." By understanding this larger system, we can get further beyond individuated consciousness, or ego, and tap into the universal intelligence of the cosmos intentionally. This understanding allows us to access a power greater than ourselves, essentially like nourishing the soil for seeding our consciousness. When supported by this greater system, you fear less, enabling you to step boldly into the unknown territory of self-creation. In Western culture, we're hyper-focused on the individual journey. Yet these archetypal forces that play out through those close to us—our friends, lovers, and family—are our deepest mirrors of ourselves, and our connection to this larger cosmic system influences us.

Within our universe is a complex system of 100 billion galaxies or more, which together form our supra-reality. This universe exists in a perpetual state of flux. Just as we breathe in and out, so does the whole universe, in a constant state of expansion and contraction. Our personal innerverse reflects this: we, too, are forever changing and evolving. When accompanied by awareness and a willingness to transcend the ego and surrender to the universal cosmic order, these states of movement and transition are opportunities to seed our consciousness with new thoughts, ideas, and ways of being. These "seeds," in turn, set a new trajectory for our existence. Psychedelics are one way to stimulate this movement, to prepare the soil in which these seeds are being planted.

This understanding of the greater cosmic order—to give context to work with psychedelics and plant medicines and the unique point that Earth is at in relationship to it—is especially relevant to our civilization at this moment in history. According to many ancient traditions, a Great Central Sun exists at the center of our galaxy, around which the Milky Way is spiraling.* This Great Central Sun is said to contain the highest concentration of intelligence, a unified field of pure consciousness. The Great Central Sun is also known as the point of singularity, the birthplace of light, referred to as Benben in ancient Egypt. I believe that this birthplace of light is where many of us go when we take a

---

*Modern astronomers believe a black hole is at the galaxy's center. No one knows for sure, but all agree there is some vast energy source that causes our galaxy to spiral in space.

breakthrough dose of 5-MeO-DMT—a place of blinding light, formlessness, all-consuming luminescence, and nonduality.

The ancient Vedism held that this Great Central Sun, or singularity point, was the reference point for historical astrological cycles or epochs. These 25,772-year cycles are the time it takes for the Earth to pass through all the degrees of the zodiac within the circling of the entire cosmos. Paramahansa Yogananda had a particular view on the cycle humanity is in now, as did his guru, Sri Yukteswar. The idea goes like this: as the cycles ascend, Earth moves closer to the Central Sun, which delivers more potent energy, the underlying force of creation, to our solar system. We are on the long trek back to a time when these creative forces will support our planetary growth. On the other hand, we are moving out of the cycle's lowest point, where Earth is furthest from the Central Sun. In this dark age, when the energy is most dense, it takes more work, often using spiritual practices, to access mystical states or transcendent consciousness. We're currently exiting this part of the cycle and so, to help us along, many spiritual practices such as chanting, kundalini yoga, breathwork, spiritual fasting, meditation, and Indigenous practices connected with psychoactive plant medicines are becoming more and more widely accessible.

In the least-dense time, which we'll be entering next, Earth will journey closer to the Central Sun of the universe again. When this happens, it will be much easier for individuals from all walks of life to become self-realized. As our galaxy moves closer to the galactic center of the universe, time quickens or can sometimes feel like it ceases to exist. The Hindus believed that during this cycle period, one soul could accomplish spiritual evolution, which would otherwise require many lifetimes, in a single lifetime. This suggests we are on track to progress greatly as a species as we enter a new Golden Age, making this an exceptional moment to traverse the deep recesses of our innerverse. But we aren't out of the woods yet. Much more darkness remains to be overcome before we enter this potent time, a time that has been foretold in many prophesies spoken by Indigenous wisdom keepers. The Kogi Kággaba, for instance, mark 2026 to be a pivotal crossing through the birth canal for humanity and Earth—just like when one crosses through the Bardo in death or a psychedelic journey—there are big changes and purges as part of this death and rebirth. Maybe the black-hole that astronomers see is actually a bardo that we will cross through someday, a belly button connected to a higher dimension.

The inherent ineffability of the innerverse, where even words fail to capture the magnificence of its flawless design—this is the truly right-brain, metaphysical part of us, and as such, it is hard to reduce it into logical, left-brain words or precise manifestations. As Lao-tzu, the founder of Taoism, stated, "The Tao that can be spoken of is not the enduring and unchanging Tao. The name that can be named is not the enduring and unchanging name." The secrecy shrouding this knowledge for ages, revealed gradually, aimed to furnish a framework to understand the ephemeral yet orderly nature of the cosmos. Whether discussing the innerverse or the broader cosmos, attempting to verbalize its essence proves futile, for its power transcends the limitations of language. While left-brained cultures may seek to rigidly define this power, it exists within intricate patterns where energy flows dynamically yet predictably, governed by an algorithmic nature. This framework represents the universal cosmic order, an interconnected system disseminating information across its vast network.

Within this cosmic symphony, each planetary body assumes a unique role, collectively guiding life through the natural cycles of creative evolution, death, and rebirth. Their harmonious interplay maintains equilibrium within the system, underscoring the intricate balance inherent to existence.

Everything is energy; therefore it is all made of the same fabric, set into motion by the great creative forces of change. Hundreds of billions of stars in the universe are emitting codes in the form of light. By codes, I mean intelligence carried within the light that is itself a seed of consciousness—when receiving it, you could call it the DNA that contains all life. The ancient Gnostic texts told that when the manifest world came into being, light flooded the cosmos from one primary source, as described earlier in the idea of the Great Central Sun. Kabbalists call this the Ensofic Ray or *Ohr Ein Sof*—the infinite light, the first primordial ray of Creation, or the original light that illuminated all things. According to the Gnostic texts, as the universe formed, this ray of light was blown apart in a "big bang," and aspects of its spiritual intelligence were distributed to form other celestial servers of consciousness, including the planets and galaxies that exist today. The concept of the big bang theory in science aligns with the idea of a primordial event that the Bwiti believe initiated the universe's expansion and evolution. It suggests that the universe began as an infinitely dense and hot state before rapidly expanding and then cooling over billions of years.

As a result of this explosion that set life into motion, each unique star and planet formed and evolved as a cosmic "server" of intelligence, each emitting a different aspect of consciousness or archetypal information. These different energies are represented within the system of astrology, with the planetary transits being used to divine how events may be influenced by the planets. As well, pyramids and temples around the world were built in alignment with the equinoxes and other significant celestial events, to allow the transmission of as much spiritual intelligence from the planets as possible during these auspicious moments.

We Are Made of Stardust

Astrology is a complex belief system that asserts the positions of celestial bodies at the time of an individual's birth can influence their personality, behavior, and life events. The birth or natal chart is a snapshot of the sky at the moment of birth and serves as the foundation for astrological interpretation. It is made up of several components, including the signs, planets, houses, and aspects, which together shape the archetypal template of someone's personality tendencies. This is all based on the placement of the stars in the sky at the exact time you were born, down to the hour.

In astrology, each of the twelve zodiac signs—Aries, Taurus, Gemini, Cancer, Leo, Virgo, Libra, Scorpio, Sagittarius, Capricorn, Aquarius, and Pisces—represents an archetypal energy and is associated with particular qualities, strengths, and weaknesses. The position of the Sun in a specific sign at the time of birth determines an individual's Sun sign, which represents the core of their personality and ego. From astrology, we learn that each planet has different characteristics and governs different aspects of human consciousness. Many systems attempt to address these planetary influences, all describing the same thing through a slightly different lens. The tarot deck, the *I Ching*, the Kabbalah's tree of life, animal totems found in many Indigenous knowledge systems, and the archetypes Carl Jung described are all different ways of understanding the universal energies present in both the cosmos and in humans. They strive to teach us about aspects of personality, behavior, and the unconscious tendencies found in every human being to varying degrees. To further illustrate this correlation, the names of the planets correspond to those of the Roman gods, and the energies attributed to each planet relate to the god it is named for. For example, Mercury is named for the Messenger God who rules communication; Venus for the Goddess of Love, representing attraction and relationships; and so on. The myths, the gods, and the planets all tell the same story: that of the archetypal and universal forces that move the cosmos.

Each planet in astrology represents different facets of an individual's life and personality. The position of the planets in the various signs and houses of the natal chart provides insight into the many aspects of that person's life, such as emotions, communication style, relationships, and career. Though I'm no astrological expert, in my studies of astrology and in giving nearly a thousand Human Design readings to others, I discovered a sophisticated programmatic algorithm that weaves the rich tapestry of the personality and relational framework itself. Each of the twelve astrological planets in our solar system influences aspects of our personality, which inform how we express ourselves. The natal chart is divided into twelve houses, which correspond to different areas of life. The houses are numbered from one to twelve, beginning with the Ascendant, or rising sign, and moving counterclockwise around the chart. Each house represents a specific domain of experience; identity, values, communication, home, creativity, work, relationships, transformation, philosophy, career, community, and spirituality. For instance, the planet Mars, connected to the astrological sign Aries, governs our power and how we might behave in business or work, while Mercury, the ruling planet of Gemini, may influence how we communicate. All this depends on the placement of the sign in our chart, as well as how it relates to other aspects of the twelve houses of the chart. For instance, if you have a lot of Libra throughout your chart, you may have a deep desire to create balance and beauty in the way you do things, or you may yearn to bring justice through advocacy. All facets of these twelve houses weave together your complex stories, your tendencies, your shadow, and your gifts. These are the golden threads that have been interlaced into a unique, one-of-a-kind pattern that makes you, you.

Aspects are the angles formed between planets in the natal chart, which indicate how different parts of an individual's personality interact and relate to one another. Aspects can be harmonious or challenging, depending on the nature of the angle and the planets involved. They help provide nuance and complexity to the astrological interpretation, revealing how different parts of someone's personality can either support or conflict with one another. These aspects can also clash with others, giving context to why some relationships have specific tension points. Tension points are opportunities to generate creative energy and spiritual growth. What would happen if you gave validation to the other, even if it's a differing view? Maybe there is something underneath it all that will reveal itself collectively, something more profound than your position or even that of the other person. For instance, many times where Joseph and I disagree, some accidental discovery occurs when we really open up to see the other's position. I have even seen that our astrological oppositions were more greatly amplified during these times. The greater lesson may have been our awareness of compassion and nurturing toward each other or the need for boundaries. The topic of the disagreement usually wasn't the core issue at all.

By looking at the interplay between the signs, planets, houses, and aspects in a birth chart, astrologers can develop a detailed and comprehensive picture of a person's archetypal template, including their strengths, weaknesses, and tendencies in various areas of life. It is important to remember, however, that astrology is a symbolic language, and its interpretations should be taken as one perspective among many when considering personality and life experiences.

In essence, astrology is simply a language that describes how each human being embodies and interacts with the greater divine order, which is influenced by spiritual, cosmic, or metaphysical intelligence personified by the different planets. Everyone has this access to all the servers of consciousness going all the way up to the Great Central Sun. The language of archetypes is the pathway that leads us there, as these archetypes allow us to connect to these different planetary servers. Ultimately, understanding archetypal influences provides a deeper awareness of how to integrate aspects of our shadows, opening a doorway to access the gifts and talents that may be latent within.

This notion of planetary aspects influencing the framework of our human lives and traumas, and shaping our personalities to some extent, is found in the research of Dr. Stanislav Grof. Over decades of research on LSD with his patients, as well as in altered states induced by endogenous DMT stimulation through holotropic breathwork, Grof found a link between astrology and the sessions he held. Not only were his ceremonies influenced by astrological events—in relation to both the date of the ceremony itself and the individual's astrological birth chart—but the individual's basic perinatal matrix also had an influence. The perinatal matrix is a four-stage process that begins in the womb at gestation and includes the process of entering the world during birth. The four stages in the perinatal matrix mirror the archetypal aspects of Neptune, Saturn, Pluto, and Uranus, as later discovered in Grof's work with Archetypal Astrologist Richard Tarnas. Within this cycle, an archetypal story arc is revealed that is often found to have been greatly affected by the astrological influences present during the process. Later life experiences and past life memories tend to mirror the experiences of one's perinatal matrix.

Simply put, our human stories are written in the cosmos, the energies represented in the stars and planets being a mediating force in each individual's unique experience of life. So are we always watching the same movie about these planetary energies interacting, just with different actors playing the characters? Joseph Campbell describes how all myths form one monomyth because they repeatedly tell the story of the human experience. They are telling your personal story too. These are the stories we keep seeing, over and over, because they relay the ongoing story of how the planets dance around the universe and how this influences us as humans.

Historical events like the First Council of Nicea and the burning of ancient texts in the Library of Alexandria have limited our modern understanding of ancient teachings and religion. The discovery of the Gospel of Thomas found buried a clay jar in a dig in 1945, in Nag Hammadi, Egypt sheds light on alternative perspectives, such as when Jesus's disciples said to him, "When will the kingdom come?" and Jesus said, "It will not come by waiting for it. It will not be a matter of saying 'here it is' or 'there it is.' Rather, the kingdom of the Father is spread out upon the earth, and men do not see it." The Gospel of Thomas was saying heaven is here, right under our noses, not some place where we go when we die. This text along with other

Gnostic texts found near a cave were thought to be hidden for 1600 years to protect them from being destroyed. What other pieces of our story could have been destroyed or rewritten? Understanding how the nature of story is embedded in every cell in our body, our microbiome, and our DNA through our ancestors, we need these original stories to heal ourselves and become whole again.

The Bwiti Fang creation story lends evidence to what the Gospel of Thomas was saying. God is male and female, all in one, the fusion of the spirits and the sexes, or creative forces, Niambi and Dinzona. This "God" created the first human couple, Nyangui and Koumba. They were what we equate to Adam and Eve, and they lived in the rainforest, which the Fang believe is Eden, heaven on Earth.

In Eden, there are two trees. One tree is the tree of the mother, tree of knowledge—acacia, or as some say, even ayahuasca, which both contain DMT. And the other tree is iboga, which is the tree of the knowledge of good and evil, which is the understanding of duality.

And just like there is symbolism in the holy communion, in Bwiti, the red represents the menstrual blood of woman, and the white represents the semen of man. In the story of communion representing the blood and body of Christ, the woman was cut out.

Essentially, our sterilized monomyth created by cutting out the stories written in the stars and ancient knowledge created the hero as our prominent story, a misconstrued story that has caused patriarchal constructs and capitalism to get out of balance. Poet and philosopher Plato warned against relying on books as the sole source of learning in *Phaedrus*:

> For this discovery of yours will create forgetfulness in the learners' souls, because they will not use their memories; they will trust to the external written characters and not remember of themselves. The specific which you have discovered is an aid not to memory, but to reminiscence, and you give your disciples not truth, but only the semblance of truth; they

will be hearers of many things and will have learned nothing; they will appear to be omniscient and will generally know nothing.

Maybe this old story will evolve as we step away from relying on books and institutions alone and rediscover our ancient roots. Perhaps the restoration of these original stories will allow us to return back to the rainforest, to Eden. Eden is very much alive, and her gifts have flowed outside the jungle to remind us of our true story. If we can't find the real story in books, we must venture into nature and the symbolic mind. Plato believed that culture wasn't about solitary book reading but about attending performances, listening to orators and poets, and watching classical actors enact tragedies. Plato argued in his critique that theater alone couldn't convey truth adequately. He contended that poets didn't merely imitate reality but rather brought it into existence through 'mimesis,' often influenced by divine possession, which played a significant role in their creative process.

These ancient stories live beyond the third dimension, in the symbolic mind, and can be accessed only by the soul and nature, and sometimes with the aids of plant medicines and psychedelics. And because the planets are always moving through space, they are always relating with each other—and therefore with life on Earth—in different ways. These interactions each contribute their energy to the pumping of the heartbeat of the cosmos, which in turn is felt within each of us. And thus the fabric of what we perceive as our reality is woven. Although they each have shadow aspects that influence the ego and our human expression of personality—in essence they can give us the antidote as they give us a greater understanding of the big picture.

We think we have free will, but the story of life and creation is the story of how these planetary bodies interact with us and through us unconsciously. We experience tension and discomfort when we insist on swimming against the natural order of these cosmic forces, often due to a calcification in the egoic template. In so doing, we miss the golden opportunities the universe offers us for our growth and evolution. But when we understand this and work to strengthen the connection between the universe and our innerverse, we can create lives that align with these forces rather than resisting them or rejecting them altogether. It is a slow journey of re-membering these stories and, through them, re-membering ourselves. But I can't tell you what your journey will be like, because it is for you to discover.

Traversing the Innerverse

As the alchemical principle reminds us, the planetary servers of consciousness transmit information at all times: "as above, so below." And navigating the inner landscape brings us into resonance with the territory of the stars. We connect to them through feeling or intuition or simply seeking guidance in a particular area. To receive their signal clearly, we must work daily to integrate life's emotional debris and traumas. As we have seen, psychedelics can help with this. We can also find clarity in nature, as the harmony of nature creates an environment that strengthens signal. When we meditate or do breathwork, we can sometimes just plug right in to the cosmos and its infinite intelligence. Dieter Duhm, founder of the intentional community Tamera in Portugal, says, "There is a world that we create, and there is the world that has created us. These two worlds must come together. This is the goal of the journey." He is speaking of the journey of self-discovery, which exists in the biofeedback loop that is created between yourself, the Earth, the beings around you, and the cosmos. This is the work of going within, and non-ordinary states and other healing tools can help us to integrate all these pieces together.

I have always been a visual thinker, so accessing my innerverse felt natural once I started to conceptualize the archetypal forces at play within me. It feels like an ancient memory: a vision of the entire cosmos as a three-dimensional map that was put together, piece by piece, seeded into my consciousness through my own practice of soul kintsugi, as well as the teachings I have studied and my experiences in medicine journeys and initiations. My work with others and the visions they share with me, in addition to things I've witnessed myself during their psychedelic experiences, reflect common threads corresponding to what I have seen myself in altered states. It took years to form this map, and many parts are still yet to be understood. The innerverse is such a vast place, yet in an instant I can focus my intention on a location and see or feel an aspect of it. Sometimes it's just a knowing, a sense of peace or under-standing. For instance, if I focus on the Bardo, the birth canal that is a pathway into the spirit world, I might see a long, dark hallway with a light glowing in the distance, or feel the tension in my body that echoes the sensation of coming out of a womb into openness and peace. In this way, I can connect with the innerverse at will, and it is now part of my being, and you can do the same.

Some of you may recognize pieces or all of this map, but continuing the practice of soul kintsugi will start to piece together the multidimen-sional, metaphysical landscape within.

The Pain Keeper

Once a women voyaged into her innerverse and met a wise old woman who showed her that there were beings on this planet who had agreed to hold the pain of humanity. The old women called them "pain keepers." She went on to tell the journeyer that she, the journeyer, was one of these pain keepers. The journeyer could then vividly draw upon a memory of her loved ones in the spirit world, standing on shore and seeing her off in her travels as she floated in a little boat, making her journey to incarnate on Earth. She felt a sense of duty as she agreed to take on this sacred mission, although there was a tinge of sadness. Moreover, she described a feeling of her individual suffering seeming small in relation to the many thousands of souls who had made that journey just like her, as there were many other boats with "pain keepers" making the trek alongside her.

I understood this pain keeper was assigned to represent the martyr archetype; it had been a pattern in the journeyer's relationships to take on other people's suffering, as she had been doing since childhood. This quality tends to be associated with the astrological influence of Virgo. Meeting this pattern in the landscape of her innerverse helped her enter a deeper place of self-acceptance and adjust her stance on how she was taking on the pain of others. She felt a profound sense of relief and emerged from the experience with renewed strength to move forward in an empowered way in her relationships. That pain keeper place is on the map of her innerverse, but it also represents a piece of herself that she has reclaimed and sealed with gold. The big takeaway for her was making this part sacred and doing it with awareness. She also was able to honor her deep sensitivity and give herself the time she needed to regroup after she was fulfilling this role.

Think about all the traumas of our separation from nature, the humiliation of all the times we missed the mark, and the suffering that results from striving for things that are not ours to hold in this life. Perhaps the greatest gift of learning to traverse the innerverse is the sense of being supported by life, Creator, or the universe—whatever you want to call it—protected and guided. All the signs and systems are in place to support us through every step on our path. Still, too often, the fear-based patterns of the egoic template prevent us from paying close enough attention and from noticing the subtle, benevolent forces that are always in communication with us. Instead, some of us repeat patterns that keep us in suffering. According to Dr. Stanislav Grof, who has over sixty years of experience in this field, "If psychiatry goes in the right direction, in my opinion, it would be working with psychedelics and using archetypal astrology as a guide." I agree. Whether our society returns to the original traditions or we create our own initiatory rituals, we must operate from a framework that allows us to reconnect to our archetypal nature, turning in to the mysteries of the universe to retrieve the map within ourselves.

Seeding consciousness, the process of awakening the part of us that is unconscious, involves learning how to understand and befriend these hidden forces, then learning how to wield them. The planetary forces live inside you—all the gods and archetypes and every myth and story ever told. All the gifts and challenges that are yours to work with in this life will be revealed to you as you journey into the realms of deep mystery, beauty, and all that is sacred. This reclamation allows you to choose how to respond, even when you may still be experiencing pain or suffering. The power to face the inner demons that create havoc within and to plant seeds in the soil of your psyche that create new neural pathways can support making more conscious choices every day. As these new roots strengthen, you will have great agency and power in your life.

Now that we have a basic framework for how the cosmic forces both shape and mirror our inner experience, the rest of this book will elucidate more clearly how to work with them consciously. The tiniest seed contains the potential to be a whole tree, but not every seed becomes one. Each human has the same potential; we embody the intelligence of the entire universe, but how we express it is down to us. The process of seeding consciousness is what allows this potential to propagate, maturate, and be fortified with strength to grow tall and someday bear fruit.

Whether you do this work with or without the aid of psychoactive medicines, committing to it will help you better navigate the realms of the psyche and integrate these experiences into something that supports or helps direct you in a meaningful way. Psychedelics are doorways to the most sacred and mystical corridors of the human experience, but these medicines alone won't bring you to what you seek. As you will discover, it is when you build a relationship over time with these universal forces and stories and humbly embrace your place in the great cosmic order that the sacred plants will work with you, through the strength of your connection to your innerverse and the seeds you have planted.

. . . .

SEEDING CONSCIOUSNESS IN PRACTICE

Star Bathing

Star bathing is a nature practice and a form of meditation in which you observe the stars while being present in your experience of receiving their light. When was the last time you sat and looked up at the night sky? Our galaxy alone is home to over 100 trillion stars, each producing energy traveling at the speed of light.

Ideally, you will find a place outside the city to practice star bathing, with less light pollution. Once you have found a suitable location, get comfortable and look up at the sky as you let your eyes adjust to the dark. Then scan the sky. Connect to the Moon. What phase is it in? Feel yourself soaking in the moonlight. What do you notice when you connect to the Moon? Maybe you will feel how it stirs up your emotions inside or awakens your intuitive capacities.

Now look for any constellations. Can you find the Big Dipper? Find Orion, which is nearby. When you look at the light of the stars making up Orion's belt, be reminded that every soul on Earth has traveled through the gateway of those stars. Does anything come up for you when you connect to this star system? You might feel a sense of home or your soul; you may even find ease in communicating with your soul in its presence. Finally, think about a question you have about your life. Is there something you need clarity on? Ask the stars what they have to say and listen. Wait for an answer to show up in your life in the coming days.

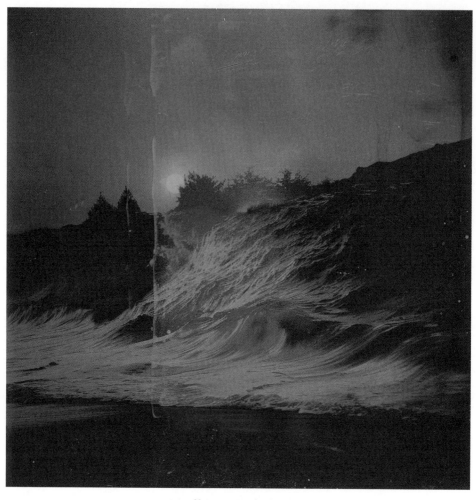

A Different Kind of Feeling

by Lela Amparo

7
Solar Eclipse
Pausing to Reclaim Our Solar Power

Someday, after we have mastered the winds, the waves, the tides, and gravity, we shall harness . . . the energies of love. Then, for the second time in the history of the world, man will have discovered fire.

PIERRE TEILHARD DE CHARDIN

Throughout human history, the celestial dance of the Sun and Moon has captivated our imaginations, leading us to seek deeper understanding of our place in the cosmos. The Sun, with its vibrant energy and life-giving warmth, embodies the essence of the masculine principles. In the creation myth from Bwiti Fang, the Sun (Kombe) and the Moon (Ngonde) are the first celestial couple. These celestial bodies are believed to have important roles in the spiritual lives of the people who adhere to this belief system.

The Sun, as the world's light and symbol of humanity, represents life, longevity, prosperity, integrity, and respect for the sacred. It serves as a guiding force for righteousness on Earth. In contrast, the Moon is associated with sanctifying spirits and purifying the hearts of humans, thereby fostering sacred and pure love.

In this chapter, we will explore how the Sun relates to the Hermetic Principle of Gender, a concept from the ancient alchemical text *The*

Kybalion, which posits that both masculine and feminine qualities are present in everything, and these complementary aspects work together to create balance and harmony. We will explore the interplay between the darkness and the light, and their influence on the human experience, seeking to understand this alchemical principle. This interplay allows the seemingly opposing forces of protons and electrons to work together to create stability in atomic structures and enables sexual reproduction in biology which depends on the union of sperm and egg to create new life. Drawing from the ancient Chinese philosophical concept of yin and yang, I'll illustrate how these complementary forces underpin the interconnectedness and interdependence of all things, including the Sun and Moon.

While the principle of gender and other hermetic principles may not provide direct scientific evidence, they offer a unique metaphor through which we can interpret the world around us. The soul itself is not gendered, and some traditions believe that we choose specific genders in our incarnation in order to learn. We have been male and female many times, so the concept of gender relates to how energy behaves in the earth realm and how to balance it. By understanding these principles, we can seed our consciousness with new perspectives, fostering a greater sense of connection and how to use these dualistic energies for creation.

Fighting with Fire

The spiritual malaise that has overtaken the Western mind—which manifests in everything from workaholism and burnout to relationship issues and lack of meaning or purpose—is rooted in an overreliance on the ego. I have shared how psychedelic journeys to the innerverse can help heal an egoic template that has become muscle-bound and calcified over time. But to truly understand why so many of us find ourselves enthralled by its power, we must take a closer look at what the ego represents from a cosmic and metaphysical standpoint. This will give us a much clearer understanding of how to balance the ego, which, when in its highest service, functions as a conduit for the intuitive whisperings of the soul.

From an astrological and archetypal perspective, the ego is an aspect of the Sun, the cosmic server of intelligence that sustains all life on Earth. The Sun animates our very being as our soul travels through the universe to be manifested in human form. The element of fire, which humans have relied upon for survival since time immemorial, is governed by the Sun. Throughout human history, the solar forces have guided us in how to master our interdependent relationship with the entire natural world. Not only have both the Sun and the fire it represents provided light, heat, and power, but the plants and trees also photosynthesize metabolized energy from the Sun and turn it directly into the caloric energy we rely upon to survive. Humans and animals literally eat sunlight in the form of the plants that feed us.

Likewise, the ego is the seat of our will and enables us to channel our solar life force energy into action. Our ability to turn solar power into action, through our outer expression, in the material realm has fueled the entire development of civilization as we know it. Seen this way, given our extensive planetary history of Sun worship, it is no surprise that civilizations have often fallen prey to ego worship, perhaps forgetting that their sun-fueled creations are expressions of a higher source. But at this point in our evolutionary history, we've been burning the metaphysical candle at both ends. Our ego-driven race to produce and consume is running rampant at full speed, allowing little room for the inner reflection necessary for us to correct course. In some ways, global warming itself can be read as a sign that we have pushed our solar-driven missions beyond the limits of what is sustainable on Earth.

Now, as scientists grapple with ways to harness the powers of the other elements to sustain life on Earth, it is vital that we do whatever we can to temper our reliance on the fiery solar urges of the ego. We must do this for ourselves as an antidote to the all-consuming nature of modern life, which has us on a collision course with existential burnout. And we must do this on behalf of our planet, as each of us does our part to help mend the tears we have collectively created in the great web of life.

To explore this transformation, one might consider the metaphor of a solar eclipse. Just as the moon momentarily obscures the blazing brilliance of the Sun, our unconscious behaviors may temporarily obscure our inner light and lead us to seek external sources of power or validation. However as the eclipse passes and the Sun's radiance returns, so too can we rediscover and realign with our inherent strength and inner guidance.

When we take time to reflect and recharge, we discover new paths toward fulfillment, safety, and support. In doing so, we shift our relationship with the Sun and the symbolic fire it represents from one of dependency or reckless pursuits to one of reverence, responsibility, and stewardship. Embracing these cosmic elemental energies with mindfulness and respect, we harness their immense creative potential, using them to illuminate our journey and empower our endeavors in harmony with the greater cosmic dance.

Elemental Fire

The key to taming the fire of the ego is to first recognize where it is out of balance. In our daily lives, an overreliance on the element of fire can manifest as burnout, exhaustion, chronic fatigue, addiction, and even premature death. Only when we take a step back and detach from the directives of an ego that is over-reliant on fire do we stand any chance of recovery and balance. But first, let's look at the role that both the Sun and fire have played throughout the ages. This will remind us that it is within our power to harness these energies to work for us rather than allowing them to consume us.

In mythology, such as the story of Prometheus, fire symbolizes the life force—the power that animates all life. Like every modern appliance known to man, all life that makes up the human and the nonhuman world is useless without plugging it in to some source of fuel. Every "machine," whether man-made or a creation of the divine, needs fire to bring it to life. We have essentially, with technology, replicated what kundalini does for all life on this planet.

In ancient times, we used fire to cook and stay warm. We then invented candles and oil lamps to light our dwellings in the absence of the Sun. Western culture went on to harness the element of fire to fuel modern civilization. It was in 1879 that Thomas Edison invented the light bulb. Before long, we could use electricity to heat our homes and cook our food, replacing the fireplace or hearth with the electric grid. One of the most important driving forces behind the Industrial Revolution of the nineteenth century was the emergence of the internal combustion engine, which gave us the ability to travel faster in trains, planes, and automobiles. Today the vast servers powering the internet—and therefore the technological revolution that has marked our passage into the new millennium—rely entirely on this same solar life force energy.

In some ways, our mastery of the solar power that lies at the center of our universe tells the story of human progress itself. Along the way, we have received many reminders that without proper stewardship, fire can destroy as quickly as it leaps into life. From devastating fires that have wiped out parts of major cities, to the Chernobyl nuclear disaster, to the wildfires which are sounding the alarm on the global climate catastrophe, we disrespect the almighty firepower at our peril. But this is precisely what has happened on an individual level, as we have externalized our relationship with fire in our ongoing quest for dominance over nature.

The source of this pattern goes back to our fathers and the absence of paternal care in modern society. Paternal care is not specific to gender but needs to be present and balanced within any individual for healthy ego formation. As noted in the chapter Individuated Consciousness, when children are raised in community, they have a more diverse range of archetypal energies to learn from, both masculine and feminine. In the early forming of the egoic template, we receive distinctive neuropatterning from our parents or caregivers, with the classically feminine embodied qualities of tenderness, sensitivity, and nurturing, and the masculine imbuing strength, provision, and protection. The role of the father, or masculine caregiver, influences the dopamine system in the brain. In its healthy state, dopamine motivates us to take action as part of the pleasure-reward system; it helps us stay alive. When this system does not develop properly, we often seek unhealthy ways to stimulate it behaviorally or through dopamine-enhancing substances, such as caffeine and stimulants. These are factors to consider in a bigger landscape of complex issues. Interestingly, iboga and San Pedro are traditionally associated with masculine energies, as they have been used to heal dopamine imbalances and are being researched for treating substance use disorders.

Both have been researched for treating substance use disorders. Some more holistic views on substance dependence might glean that we may be unconsciously seeking the external love or support of the masculine, which we have the capacity to generate within ourselves once we have formed a proper archetypal understanding of it.

On both a collective and an individual level, our reliance on fire as the paternal source of safety and support that we never received as children has made us like moths drawn to a flame, flying closer and closer to the light until it consumes us. Our addiction to the element of fire lies at the root of much of the hyper-masculine pattern of self-destruction that plagues Western culture. This addiction has led us to an over-extraction of the Earth's resources. Fire carries a yang, or masculine, quality that fuels creativity, confidence, and action when it is used wisely. But when we use our firepower to control others or seek power outside ourselves, it creates a state of war within and around us. Our creative drive, and the actions this inspires us to take, are no longer coming from a place of divine inspiration but from the fear and the unprocessed shadow that expresses from our egoic template.

This expression of elemental imbalance shows up when we take action from the mind without turning inward to consult intuition, as communicated to us by our other emotions or senses. Intuition is the realm of the lunar energy of the Moon, which exists in the cosmos as a natural and vital counterpoint to the Sun. The Sun and Moon are not planets; they are luminaries. A luminary is a source of light or a teacher. When we look to the Sun and Moon, they remind us of the forces beyond our control; they center us in humility and reverence for something bigger than ourselves. This is why both are so close to us and an ever-present part of our lives. Both remind us that every day is a death and rebirth. The Sun is a masculine archetype, and the Moon is a feminine archetype. The Sun is fire, and the Moon is water. One is no less or more important than the other. They each represent a dynamic part of our complex innerverse, the inner expression of these archetypal energies. When one is out of balance, it affects the entire system, as they work together harmoniously. What's most important is the integration of both aspects within ourselves.

And suppose we have become over-reliant on solar power for our survival, keeping the lights on at all times and allowing little space to reside in the unknown places of the dark. In that case, we have equally lost our ability to tune in to the watery, soulful, lunar energies that regenerate us and bring meaning to our lives (which we will examine in more depth in the following chapter).

As such, healing our relationship to fire means bringing Sun and Moon back into balance and learning how to live in respectful stewardship of the solar element once again—both externally and within ourselves. Psychedelics and other plant medicines offer us an opportunity to "unplug" from the solar grid and reflect on how we have become slaves to the egoic fire that burns within. With proper guidance on these journeys, we are shown ways to harness our own solar power—our creative life force energy—to nourish the seeds that are being sown in our consciousness rather than scorching the very soil they are rooted in. During these initiations, we can reconnect with the unseen and often undervalued lunar energies in powerful and undeniable ways.

Meanwhile, as long as we are preoccupied with seeking power externally we will not see the value of taking the journey to our innerverse to attune our egoic template and integrate all our inner exiled parts. But this is exactly where we plug into our true power. Learning to balance fire with water allows the seeds in our consciousness to flourish and grow, so we'll begin to live from a place of creative self-expression rooted in our intuition's guidance. And we will quickly discover that the fresh green shoots sprouting up can nurture and sustain us, just as surely as the plants that deliver the Sun's energy.

Solar Powered

Part of the work of harnessing the solar energies safely and productively is gaining a full understanding of the role that this energy plays in our lives. Let us look back to the heavens for guidance on this. Every day, when the Sun rises once again, we embrace the birth of a new day, a new life. Before electricity became so prevalent, our ancestors lived in alignment with the rhythms of the Sun and the Moon. We rose as the Sun rose on the horizon, glowing and warming the land. We went to rest as it disappeared, revealing the nighttime veil of stars cast across the sky and the moon waxing and waning through its cycles. These cosmic movements of light and dark are imprinted into our physiology, managing what are known as circadian rhythms in our bodies. These rhythms affect our hormonal balance and melatonin production, regulating our sleep at night and our energy levels throughout the day—just one of many ways the movement of cosmic bodies impacts the experience of our innerverse.

As with all the stars in the cosmos, the Sun emits light. Light is made up of photons, which in turn are made up of waves of electromagnetic radiation. This light contains the information, or cosmic code, that animates us and all life. The light from our Sun feeds us prana, as the Hindu philosophers refer to it, or chi, as the Chinese named it. We can think of this simply as our life force, and it is the very same force as the kundalini that I introduced in the chapter on ego death.

At certain times of the year, the Earth is closer to the Sun. During these times, we are better positioned to "charge up" on the Sun's power; the ancients believed these could be times of great spiritual advancement. The word "enlightened" reflects our special relationship with light. Ancient civilizations, from the people of Kemet to the Mayans, built temples designed to help us connect to this powerful cosmic body for heightened awareness and manifestation. They sought this awareness through prayers, ceremonies, and rituals that paid reverence to the power of the Sun.

In addition, the Sun is associated with the metal gold, representing our highest creative self-expression in the practice of inner alchemy. As we have seen, the element of fire is the earthbound equivalent of the Sun. And as fire represents power, so does the Sun. The question, for anybody who is invested in mastering this power and transmuting the base energies of existence into creative gold, is what we will choose to do with the power that we've been given in this life. Fire is our prana, chi, or life force; it provides us with the impetus and energy to take action on the thoughts and ideas that blossom in our consciousness. These actions are most aligned with our soul's purpose—that is, with our individual role within the web of life—when we can infuse our actions with the directives of our emotional body, our inner moon. We practice this when engaging with any sort of divination or journeywork. Rather than simply using the force of our will to push through life, we take a moment to intuit what actually *needs* to be done. That way, we conserve our storehouses of chi to maintain our vitality.

Questions we can ask when learning to direct our solar power responsibly and effectively might be: Is this the right time to be doing this thing? If not, what is the best use of my time? The answers will present themselves when we can quiet the demands of the willful ego (Sun) and tune in to the soft voice of the soul (Moon). Approaching our actions in this way reminds us that there is always time to create and work, and time for rest. We remember that working through exhaustion causes mistakes, accidents, misalignment to our authentic selves and makes us susceptible to illness. Resting, pausing, stopping to feel what your body needs, and taking time to connect with yourself and the universe—outside in nature if you can—brings inspiration that makes the work more efficient when you return to it, recharged from within. Moving through the world is like breathing, in and out, a pattern that gives us the space to pause and orient ourselves.

Solar Power Struggles

Through consistent practice and discipline, we learn to work with the fire element so it doesn't burn out of control in our lives. This means recognizing that with each decision we make and each action we take, we have the choice to be directed purely by the ego or to incorporate the subtle, intuitive wisdom of the soul. When we stop to check in with our soul before taking action, we open the doorway of possibilities that can often lead to grace, blessings, and love. We can find a metaphor for this within the chakra system, where the Sun corresponds to our solar plexus, the seat of our free will and the domain of the inner child. In its healthiest form, the joyful self-expression of a child is always supported and held by the loving guidance of their parents. In the context of our relationship to the cosmic forces that created us, the Sun, our "father," supports us in the world, while the Moon, our "mother," is the fount of all nurturance and care. Safely held by the energies of both these luminaries, we are free to dance, act, play, and create—we are free to live!

But the Sun can scorch, too. Sun creates, but it also destroys. We see this duality in the solar plexus chakra, which governs our anger, rage, creativity, and joy; it holds opposite sides of the same coin. Creation opposes destruction. Joy opposes rage.

Anger is an important aspect of sovereignty. Often arising as a sign that our boundaries have been crossed, it is wielded by the warrior within, representing our will to live. This primal aspect recalls the animal part of us that had to kill or fend off predators to survive. But in our modern world, where survival is not dependent on physical force, our anger is often misplaced, denied, or suppressed. When we give presence to our anger, it alchemizes to grief, and fire becomes water in the form of tears. Part of stewarding our solar power is acknowledging our anger and accepting it as part of us. When anger arises, you can ask it why it is present, if this is not immediately evident. We can use our breath to feel the anger or even create the space for a pause, a rest from anger's intense force, consciously breathing into the parts of the body where we feel its fire to help move the energy through deep, conscious inhalation and exhalation. Specifically, when there is a lot of fire, open mouth exhalation will dispel heat. You will feel the heat in your breath as you push it out of your body. We can shake our bodies to allow the heat to come to the surface and be dispersed. We can scream, moan, yell, or dance, allowing the fire to move freely through, rather than burning up inside. When these emotions accumulate, it is important to use practices such as shaking, yelling, releasing into a punching bag, or receiving some grounding somatic bodywork to allow the energy to disperse in a way that does not harm yourself or others.

Ambition is another aspect of fire or solar power that can become out of balance. Ambition is fueled by desire. It is the force that animates our creative energy; like a flame, it reaches upward and outward, shining brighter and hotter as it burns. We have much to thank this inner flame for—it drives us to create, collaborate, dream big, and construct our realities. But the shadow aspect of ambition is attachment to desired outcomes or fixating too intensely on a goal that may not be aligned with our soul's purpose or may lead to other outcomes. This can set us up for constant striving, feelings of failure, and even grief if we lose or never win what we desire. It can also keep us in a perpetual rat race of accumulation and achievement, resulting in an unconscious need for material attainment to feel a sense of meaning, safety, or motivation and putting our happiness in the future rather than the present moment.

It's easy to see parallels between unchecked ambition and addictive tendencies, which both result from an imbalance in our solar energies. Addiction manifests as constant craving and seeking outside of ourselves in an attempt to nourish what feels like a gaping void within. Many people seek to address this void with anesthetizing or stimulating drugs to numb the pain or try to fill the emptiness with fame and external validation. Addictions to money and "success" are common in the West, as we mistake the ease that comes with material abundance for true peace of mind or safety. In the same way, addictions to sex and relationships may unconsciously be our attempts to feel worthy, seen, and whole. And we see this same energetic signature in corporate greed, which destroys landscapes and communities to scratch an insatiable itch of "not-enoughness." When in truth what the ego truly craves, wants, and desires is to be reconnected with the great web of life which grounds this imbalanced energy. Addiction echoes ceaselessly, resonating a deep longing to the soul—a primal call for attention, care, and love.

Much of the trauma of the domesticated human—the agricultural human, the sedentary human—is due to our separation from our instincts, our intuition, and the nurturing lunar energies within. Many lifetimes of ancestral trauma from our forebears who starved or experienced war and suffering have accumulated in Western epigenetic imprints. Our fears of never being or having enough and the fiery overdoing and overconsumption that stem from this are rooted in a complete severing from our inner guidance system—the cosmic innerverse, through which we may reawaken to our unending connection to all that exists. This reconnection can enable us to return to fully trusting in life once again and to heal this ancestral trauma so it is not passed down to future generations. What would it take for you to be willing to examine the parts of yourself that are pushing with excess flame toward your wants and desires? How might you instead open yourself up, to listen and intuit what your heart and soul truly need? The egoic programming of Western society has interfered with our ability to discern these needs. But the practice of seeding consciousness reminds us that the answers always lie within. The practice points us inside to clear out the backlog of stuck emotions and old programming in the psyche, which has been causing us to externalize our needs or seek to control our lives in unhealthy or imbalanced ways.

Only a lunar process of going within can resolve our solar power struggles—that is, by becoming more intimately acquainted with our subconscious mind, intuition, heart's desire, emotions, memories, and deeper motivations. Otherwise we are like a donkey chasing the proverbial carrot on a stick, precariously situating our salvation and happiness close enough to see but never close enough to truly reach. The fiery thrill of the chase might give us a high, but reaching our goals holds little nourishing substance or satisfaction. It could even be that depression and other mental malaise that one might experience could be nature's safety measure, putting the brakes on when you are about to run off a cliff, or the sign of deep burnout.

Before introducing psychedelics into the mix, this lunar process can begin with asking these questions, rather than succumbing to the unconscious urges: What is it that I need? What is my purpose? What is my inner guidance or intuition directing me toward? What am I really hungry for? Keep asking these questions every day, even if it takes months. Get quiet and listen. Instead of seeking the answers, allow them to come to you. They may come in the most subtle of ways, to ensure that you are truly listening for them—as a sign, through a friend, in nature, or even in a book. Take each step slowly. Contemplate and reflect in a journal throughout the process. Let go of any goal or attachment to any end result. Slow down and just feel for a moment. Allow the space for your inner self to unravel. Taking this time without attachment to the result is an act of self-love. Over time, you may notice a filling of your cup, a greater sense of fulfillment without having to do or obtain.

Stewarding the Fire Within

We seek fire externally because most of us are starved of vital cosmic energies. But you will never drill enough oil or extract enough gold to fulfill this deep yearning and hunger. Over the years, I have worked with many people to shift their relationship to their solar power and choose ways to direct their creativity and life force energy to light them up instead of burning them out. People experiencing solar power struggles often come to me in the grip of a career crisis. They are successful, but they have lost all sense of meaning in their work and they have either crashed and burned or they are just going through the motions.

When aiming to rebalance your inner flame, the first place to look is at any habitual practices you're using to medicate feelings of overwhelm and exhaustion that may stem from an imbalance of solar energies. If these patterns are depleting or extractive in any way, we work to replace them with habits that nurture and support the system. Many people drink a glass or two of wine to calm down after a solar-centric workday, followed by a strong cup of coffee to kick-start the system again in the morning. For others, overeating is a way to feel nurtured and supported, or to deal with emotions that have gone unprocessed in the constant churn of productivity. But these are Band-Aid alternatives to real time spent on self-care. Relying on stimulating substances is like fighting fire with fire. What is really needed is to learn how to nurture oneself from within.

Balancing the Solar with the Lunar

One woman I've worked with closely for many years owns a company in the hospitality industry. When she first came to me, the business was wearing on her. She socially and regularly drank as part of her job, was experiencing mood swings and poor sleep, and was noticing her overall inspiration to participate in life dwindle. My first recommendation was that she shift to a more plant-based diet as a way to alkalize the acidity of too much fire, from a stressful lifestyle and lots of alcohol, meat, cheese, and other rich foods. I also suggested she stop drinking alcohol completely, to help cleanse her body and give her overworked liver a break. The liver holds anger, the emotion of fire. When the liver is under stress, it can cause imbalances in emotions. I recommended she try blue lotus as a tea to help her relax and feel more creative at night. She also used CBD and GABA to help her turn off her active brain and sleep, rather than drinking alcohol to shut off her overstimulated brain.

Regarding plant medicines, she had expressed interest in microdosing with psilocybin mushrooms. Microdosing is a gentler way to feel a connection to the psychoactive plant medicines. In our solar, doing-obsessed world, it has come to be considered a "performance-enhancing" practice—because it helps open new neural pathways, connecting us to our intuition and creativity. But this is deceptive; using the medicines in this way actually serves to slow us down and connect us more deeply to the present moment and our intuition. Yes, we might have better ideas under the influence of sub-perceptual doses of psychedelics, but we won't necessarily "get more done." I think it can be used in context with intentional practice rather than purely to optimize. I see them more as integrative than generative, although in slowing us down they help create new neural pathways and can be emotionally healing.

For this woman, I felt that microdosing would support her, along with her daily practices of spending time in nature, doing yoga, and connecting with art. These activities are more yin—meaning feminine, regenerative, or Moon-centered—and so they helped her bring balance to her fiery yang, masculine lifestyle of doing and being productive. Microdosing can nourish the soil for the seeds of consciousness we've planted in deeper journeywork and can support the integration of psychedelic experiences. It can also help one create the space within to step back and observe one's patterns and choose to respond differently if needed. Patterns of emotional reactivity are a sign of overreliance on the Sun, as a build-up of unacknowledged emotions can be overwhelming when there is no lunar release valve.

I also guided this woman in a lunar fast, during which she consumed only juice and light teas over four days while tapping into the four elements and the archetypal energies they represent. The purpose of fasting is to learn to transcend our desires, which are often driven by the subconscious mind or by parasites such as candida that feed on sugars in the body and send signals to the brain telling us to eat things that harm our well-being. Fasting "resets" the body, and studies by the University of Southern California Longevity Institute have recently shown that three days of fasting can strengthen the immune system. When done properly, taking the right precautions, fasting can be more effective than plant medicine work in certain cases. I will mention, as a caveat, that anytime fasting does have medical risks, I always advise consulting a doctor to ensure there are no preexisting health issues that could make it contraindicated.

I asked the woman what her intention was entering into the cleanse. She said that she wanted to receive insight and clarity in her life and purge old things that no longer fit in the new life she was shaping for herself. Following the cleanse, she felt a great sense of direction and received an understanding of how to manage the fire within. Much of her drive was connected to pain from past grief, including her husband's health and a fire that had destroyed her family home. The loss was devastating for her. She was also fearful of Covid-19 and the constant forest fires around her that threatened her. The fasting showed her far more than her work with the psychedelics did; it was through taking this time to rest and reset that she could see the true value of her creativity and potential. Overall, it has led her to a more prayerful and intentional lifestyle with regular time dedicated to herself to process emotions. She is more grounded, more trusting of life in potentially threatening or triggering situations, and can gracefully navigate through it all. The fear that drove her no longer has such a tight grip on her.

As part of her ongoing commitment to stewarding her solar power, I encouraged her to get regular somatic bodywork, as good bodywork can help you inhabit your body more fully and freely. In my opinion, somatic body work from a trauma informed practitioner is one of the most integrative modalities with spiritual work to help move any residual blocked energy in the body and ground the experiences with psychedelics. I also recommended a regular yin yoga practice to help

release any stress that was being held in her body. These simple "lunar"
practices proved instrumental in allowing her to create boundaries for
herself, enabling her to do more of the things that nurture her and
bring her joy. She has even been inspired to invest in some healing
tools, such as crystal sound bowls and a medicine drum, which she
enjoys playing. Above all, she has remembered the value of slowing
down, which has been instrumental in healing her solar power balance.

I built a water wheel many years ago with Marshall Jack, Golden Eagle, of the Washoe Tribe of California and Nevada. Golden Eagle shared, "the bear says if you use your own energy to climb the mountain you will grow old." The wise bear uses energy from the mountain to climb it. Bears are quite large, and they are masters of using rest, hibernation, and abiding by the laws of nature so they don't waste away with the immense energy requirements needed to maintain their size. This is the same concept that biodynamic farmers use to grow abundant crops: harnessing the power of nature rather than working against it. This is a regenerative way of looking at our actions and energy, rather than just keeping the lights on all the time.

We must come into sacred relationship to fire so that it doesn't destroy us. What rebalancing adjustments can you make for yourself as you turn your attention to stewarding your inner fire? What things can you eliminate, and what boundaries can you create for yourself to create space to support the seeds you are planting in your consciousness flourish and grow?

We can begin to heal our relationship with the element of the Sun by literally rekindling a sacred bond with fire. This can be done with a candle, or an actual fire if there is a safe place available for you to do so. Ceremonies from many corners of the world, like that of the Hopi of northern Arizona who keep a sacred fire that has been burning for generations, center on fire as a symbol of the ball of fire at the center of our solar system. When we use fire ceremonially, we are reminded that while the flame warms and enlivens us, it also helps us to burn away what no longer serves us. It is a bridge to the spirit world. In Bwiti initiations, a fire always burns to protect participants from negative spirits and to clear negative energies released during the cleansing process.

· · · · · · · · · · · · · ·

SEEDING CONSCIOUSNESS IN PRACTICE

Fire Ceremony

To enact your own fire ceremony, start your fire in an intentional and sacred way. Be mindful of everything—how you arrange the kindling, the placement of the logs, how you light the fire, and how you tend to the flames. When I light a fire, I remember this advice from a Mēxica abuela (grandmother): If you try to light the fire with your mind, it will go out. Light it with your heart, and it will burn bright. You can also consider offering something to the fire—it can be a pinch of tobacco or even a sacred song.

During ceremonies that I facilitate, inspired by the Bwiti tradition, we begin by connecting around the fire. To establish this connection, each participant introduces themselves by stating their full name, their mother's full maiden name, and their father's full name. Once this connection is established, we then ask the fire for healing and guidance. This practice can be performed using either a candle or a fireplace. As you focus on the flame, observe how it responds to your inquiries. Does it sway to the left or right? Does it form distinctive shapes? Pay attention to the logs and embers as they burn; they may take on the shape of an animal, or the arrangement of the logs may convey a particular pattern. Consider what these manifestations signify to you. Direct your attention back to the fire and allow yourself to become absorbed in its flames, gradually feeling your own presence fade away. In this moment, how do you perceive the fire communicating with you? Listen closely to the crackling, popping, and hissing and the movement of the wind. Do certain sounds coincide with specific thoughts or feelings? Perhaps the fire is drawing your attention to something significant.

The fire also serves as a receptacle for offerings and confessions. Offer something that burdens your heart to the flames. For instance, you might write down your fears on a piece of paper and then burn them in the fire as a symbolic act of release. Through our connection to the fire, we are linked with the spirit of fire itself. By nurturing this connection, the fire can provide support in various aspects of our lives. Simply by gazing into the flames, we may notice that they have the power to dispel dark energies that cause confusion and fear. Personally, I often beseech the fire for protection and the dissolution of my illusions, ignorance, and distortions.

Cultivating awareness within our consciousness allows us to scrutinize and challenge unconscious behaviors, beliefs, and patterns. This process is particularly pertinent in our efforts to rebalance our relationship with the Sun and fire. By turning inward and heightening our awareness of our thoughts and emotions, we can disrupt old patterns in our relationship with fire. Just as fertile soil is essential for the germination of seeds, our minds must be receptive for this process to unfold.

As a society, rekindling the metaphorical fire can have profound effects. Gathering around this symbolic fire can foster empathy and understanding as we share our stories and momentarily transcend our differences and divisions. At its most profound level, fire embodies the accumulated wisdom passed down through generations of humanity—a wisdom that must be nurtured and protected. Many indigenous cultures maintain perpetual fires tended by their medicine people, symbolizing the potency of their prayers. These prayers are akin to the warmth and light emanating from a hearth, connecting the current generation to their ancestors and future descendants. The responsibility of safeguarding this knowledge is entrusted to those who demonstrate commitment, respect, and responsibility. It is indeed a great honor to receive this mantle. Through these simple yet profound practices and our relationships with the elements, we can invite and receive abundant blessings into our lives.

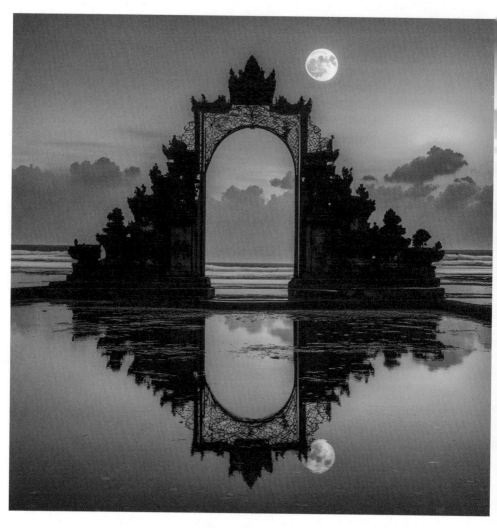

Moon Empowered

by Tricia Eastman

8
Moon Empowered
Restoring Inner Harmony

His journey is not a reflection of the moon. It is the moon itself. He is not separate from this quest. It is his dharma, his path, his voice. It is not a bead on a mala, not a veil to remove. It is the cooperation of elements, the marriage of spirit and flesh. It is the shadow of faith, the reflection of being. It is the full metaphor. It is all there is.

THOMAS LLOYD QUALLS

In the summer of 2022, China discovered a helium-3 crystal on the Moon that has the potential to provide fuel for limitless energy using fission technology. This transparent crystal has a width comparable to a single strand of human hair. Changesite-(Y), the name given to the phosphate mineral by the Beijing Research Institute of Uranium Geology, pays homage to Chang'e, the legendary Chinese Moon goddess. A discovery like this might challenge our typical conceptualizations of energy being associated with a solar source—even fossil fuels contain the solar energy captured in ancient plants. However, it is resonant with the lunar principles in alchemy and may point us toward discovering new non-fire types of power. This is also true within the process of seeding consciousness: when we tap into the energies of the

Moon, we can generate energy like a vortex, seemingly from nothingness. Bringing our relationship with solar energies back into balance is essential for our times and our survival as a species. The essence of this balance is learning to unplug from external sources of power and turn our reflection and pursuits inward. This is where we meet our lunar essence, which we experience as our emotions, sixth sense, and intuition. By the power of the Moon, our oceans and rivers rise and fall, like the motions of a person breathing, reminding us that each life-giving inhale must be balanced with a soothing, restorative exhale. The Moon is a regenerative resource that can provide life and vitality when tapped into. This is where the seeds are gestating in the soil, nurtured by the waters.

Take the example of biodynamic farming, an ancient practice of planting and growing food, which is largely based upon seeding growth around the lunar cycles. New seeds are sown, and plants are pruned when the moon is in a descending cycle, to support growth. Planting seeds into the soil just before the new moon helps create the proper conditions and cycles for them to sprout, and then harvest times occur as the moon is in an ascending phase. The descending phase is when nature breathes in, drawing in growth below the surface of the Earth, reflective of the inner or subconscious work; and the ascending phase is the out breath. Biodynamic farming and other ancestral practices, such as ceremonies use the moon cycles to encourage abundant crops and protect them from the harm of insects or other disasters that ancients believed were a product of being out of balance with nature. You can see how nature is supporting you as it breathes in and out in this way. It seems absurd for our society to rely completely on inefficient fuel sources that lead to scarcity due to their limits, and essentially work against the forces of nature when we rely on them alone. When seeding our consciousness, we work with and alongside nature according to the natural cycles, using both the Sun and Moon in balance.

In astrology, the Moon is connected to water, the element that soothes and calms our inner and outer fire. Within the universal order, the Moon is the luminary that presides over our innerverse. This luminous entity represents our emotional body as the seat of our inner wisdom (literally "insight"), our capacity for introspection, and our connection to the ancestors. "Aluna," as the Kogi Kággaba refer to her, is also the teacher of cycles; her monthly waxing and waning are a reminder that everything within the realm of our experience undergoes cycles of birth, death, and reincarnation. In both literature and certain spiritual traditions such as Bwiti, we see the Moon representing the deepest waters of our psyche or subconscious mind—the place which we enter when we "learn to die" as we boldly travel the innerverse and engage with the work of attuning the ego. Connecting with the Moon helps us to cool down and process whatever the Sun has brought boiling to the surface, allowing for integration, reflection, and insight.

The insights we gain from our journeys to the watery lunar realm are the literal "seeds" that are planted in the black soil of the subconscious, or nigredo, to be transformed into solar-powered, creative gold that flourishes into behaviors rooted in awareness. These seeds help us to get clear on what needs to be planted and what has already taken root in the soil of the psyche. It makes sense that most of society wants to avoid this lunar/inner place, as it can be messy, dark, and uncomfortable, and can show us things we don't want to see about ourselves. Also, most modern psychology doesn't scratch the surface of these aspects of the psyche, as one must be in an altered state in order to access what lies far beneath conscious awareness. You can access these states through meditation, hypnosis, sound healing, breathwork, and psychoactive plant medicines or psychedelics. Modern-day talk therapy provides ways of coping with the effects of any trauma residing in the subconscious, but the actual wound is buried in the psyche like a landmine that one will stumble upon eventually, causing destruction and havoc in one's life. Through the processes outlined in this book, we can, over time, disarm these landmines and safely integrate them into the psyche.

Modern psychology has gotten one thing right: 95 percent of the human operating system is sourced from the subconscious soil. Seeding consciousness is an ongoing process of refinement and awareness around what exactly is being planted, rooted, and cultivated within the subconscious. We can't even gaze into the psyche without a key to unlock the doorway of the subconscious, the realm represented by the Moon. But in the West, an overemphasis on the solar/yang/active/conscious mind—and the productive, materialist ideals it promotes—has atrophied our ability to enter the lunar realm. As such, it is on us to consciously reestablish our lost connection to Mother Moon, and in doing so to come back home to our whole selves. It is critical that we balance the solar and lunar energies within ourselves and keep this balance strong, as the moment we get out of balance, the inertia and patterning of the unconscious will come back in and attempt to override the work that we've done.

The Dark Side of the Moon

In the Kogi language, *Aluna* literally translates literally as "Moon," but in the Kogi cosmovision, it is also applied to the metaphysical concepts represented by the glowing celestial pearl. The Kogi mamos, who are selected through divination, spend at least nine years in a cave or hut to cultivate their intuition and internal light by connecting with Aluna. This is their initiation to serving as Guardians of Earth. Elsewhere, the abuelas of Mēxica in Mexico perform the Moondance ritual to connect to the wisdom of the feminine Moon. The tradition is linked to Coyolxāuhqui, the Aztec lunar goddess who was torn apart by her brother Huītzilōpōchtli, the Aztec god of war. He cast her head to the sky, where it became the Moon, and the rest of her body was scattered into the heavens. Coyolxāuhqui is a reminder of the deconstruction and reconstitution that happens in the cycles of life and death. The Moondance ritual is a sacred rite for women only. In this tradition The Moondancer is said to develop shape-shifting abilities over time, becoming what's known as a *nahual*. This mythical figure is believed to harness the qualities of animals and elements through a deep connection with nature's forces. These examples remind us to look to the power that we, too, can gradually reclaim when we build our own relationship with the Moon.

The Moon is revered as a source of great wisdom and power in ancient cultures. So why is Aluna so disempowered and denigrated in the West? The answer to this is multifaceted, like the Moon herself. The elusive, ever-transforming face of the Moon lends itself to motifs of mystery and the great unknown; her very nature is uncertainty, a quality that is anathema to egoic Western ideals of linear progress and rationality. Indeed, the full moon is the origin of the term *lunacy** and has inspired fables of frenzied human metamorphoses from man into wolf. Stories of werewolves howling at the Moon tell of deep-seated fears of our more primal nature and the threat that our emotions and unconscious desires pose to the linear order of the status quo.

On an individual level, those disconnected from our inner selves are afraid, even terrified, to journey into the subconscious and connect with this part of ourselves for fear of what one might encounter. Some people experience sheer terror when they embark on a psychedelic journey, due to backed-up emotions and traumas—even more reason to unplug from solar consciousness and plunge into the lunar depths. Astrological mythology holds a clue as to where this terror originates,

*See John Swan's *The Speculum Mundi*, which describes lunacy as a malady whose progression mirrors the phases of the Moon. Nonnus's "Dionysiaca" further explores this theme, asserting, "I, alongside Bacchus, govern frenzied madness. I am the lunar deity of Bacchic rites, not solely for my celestial orbit through the months, but also for my authority over insanity and stimulation of lunacy. I am the Bacchic Mene, not alone because in heaven I turn the months, but because I command madness and excite lunacy."

specifically, the legend of Black Moon Lilith. Representing the apogee, or the furthest point from Earth along the Moon's orbit, Black Moon Lilith governs our most primitive behaviors. Wherever this point shows up in your astrological birth chart reveals your most hidden side and the place in your life where you have become disempowered due to the primal parts of your nature having been suppressed. In effect, Lilith represents our personal and cultural shadow side. But these shadowy parts are exactly where we must venture if we are to bring awareness to the unconscious patterns, behaviors, and beliefs that will otherwise keep sabotaging us from behind the veil.

Many are so afraid of the dark, so enthralled with the clarity and certainty of the light, that we have created monsters from our own shadows, clinging to what is known, even when it threatens to destroy us, rather than stepping into the unknown. But, as Carl Jung put it, "The shadow is a living part of the personality and therefore wants to live with it in some form. It cannot be argued out of existence or rationalized into harmlessness." These aspects of self, when left untended, will lurk in the dark corners, waiting for the opportune moment to strike. For the sake of ourselves and those around us, we must either disarm them by integrating them or be prepared with tools ready for when they rise to the surface. When we proactively get deep into the shadow, we can identify these hazards before they create problems in our daily lives. Over time, and with regular nurturance, the grumpy exiled monster that we created can be integrated or at least tamed, its wildness no longer destructive but a source of unbridled self-expression, creativity, and metaphorical "drunken" surrender.

This fear of the dark, the territory of the Moon, is the root of the oppression of the feminine principle, which exists in people of every gender expression. Ancient folklore recognized Lilith as the first woman, created by God as Adam's equal. Rejected by him on account of her strong-willed nature, she precedes the biblical Eve, created of Adam as his companion, though she was often blamed for initiating the fall from the grace in the garden. As such, Lilith represents the archetype of the dark feminine, personifying the psyche's rejected aspects or rogue parts. On a mythological level, she is the original martyr, just as the fall of the Gnostic feminine goddess Sophia, which began from her being misunderstood, has led to a deep wounding to the balance of power between the Sun and Moon. The goddess never "fell," she materialized as earth, matter and mother being one in the same. This myth also exists in the Bwiti Fang tradition, but instead of the apple tree, the tree is the large bush *Tabernanthe iboga*—the tree of knowledge of good and evil, more appropriately described as the tree of duality.

For the Bwiti, iboga is a source of wisdom, spiritual insight, and deep healing. When consumed, the iboga root bark provokes intense visions and introspective experiences, allowing users to confront their fears, traumas, and negative patterns. Bwiti practitioners believe that iboga can facilitate communication with ancestors and spiritual beings, providing guidance and knowledge on how to live a harmonious and fulfilling life. In the Bwiti story told by the Fang, the Eve-like figure named Nyangui takes the iboga and becomes aware of reality's dualistic nature. Good and bad really only live inside us when we desire something or when we reject it. This very duality inhabits our nervous systems. This is the wound of separation, which we create within or can choose to unify by seeding our consciousness. Recall the character Neo in the movie *The Matrix*, who takes the red pill and is made deeply aware of the Matrix and exposed to the harsh realities of suffering, while being simultaneously awakened to great power within himself.

The feminine (Moon) and masculine (Sun) principles working *together*, in nature, in society, and within us as individuals, are the very essence of the creative cycles of life. "Birthing" anything new begins by venturing into the dark of the womb space and potentially facing things that are painful and scary. It means going into the shadow, as presided over by the inner moon, and calling on our Sun power to bring awareness to the unconscious patterns that are keeping us stuck. Interestingly, the more we sit with something and ask it questions to understand what it is—rather than what we think it is, or what it was for us in the past—the more we bring light to it. It may change without us needing to actually "do" anything. In essence, we can compost our trauma by giving it our attention. Suppose the cure for overreliance on our solar power is to honor and harmonize our lives and actions with the mysterious workings of the inner moon. In that case, we must seek this harmony first and foremost, to integrate our separate and exiled parts back into the whole.

We fear our shadow so deeply, yet the demons, ghosts, and other ghouls of the underworld, subconscious, or shadow are really the janitors of the universe. These energies are here to clean up what is not in harmony with life, that which is decaying and stagnant. Even death itself is beckoning us toward a new life. When our "demons" chase us in the form of depression, anxiety, or repetitive negative thoughts, it is a reminder that something within us needs to embrace change or that it is time to let go of something. These forces are not here to hurt us but to shape us, to point us inward and process or "clean up" any blockages that are being acted out in our daily lives. This is what we are doing when we connect with our inner moon: cleaning our own house and receiving directions to move forward on the right course, away from stagnation or death. We can't just keep pushing forward like wounded, limping soldiers; we need access to reclaim our original story and with it our power to heal. For this, we must make time to restore ourselves to get clarity and find our center, as our Mama Moon would urge us to do.

Our mothers are the first to teach us about the Moon, when we are suspended in the womb. In utero, we are fully dependent upon the substance of the maternal source in a watery abyss. As we emerge into the world, the mother nurtures us and tends to us with gentleness to soothe our cries. Ideally, the mother's intuition helps her know what her baby needs, as this budding life cannot communicate with words. The connection and bonds we forge with our mothers both supports our development and catalyzes the release of serotonin and bonding hormones such as oxytocin and prolactin in them. But many who play this important maternal role in the modern era are forced to return to jobs and productivity—to enter into the solar realms—before the infant fully develops the capacity to self-soothe through difficult emotional states. New mothers who live in stressful environments or have too much of their own trauma can be impaired in their capacity to provide the nurturing support that a newborn child needs to effectively complete this vital process.

This can lead children to experience anxiety, sleep problems, digestive problems, and depression later in life. Breastfeeding also plays a key role since there is such a deep association between emotional self-regulation—mediated through the gut and serotonin pathways—and maternal bonding. This mother-and-baby relationship sets the stage for healthy serotonin production later in life. However, the relationship between early bonding and serotonin function is complex and still being studied. Proper serotonin function is important for overall emotional health. Serotonin receptors, specifically 5-HT_{2A} has been linked to peak mystical experiences, typically induced by ingestion of DMT-containing substances.

Walking on the Moon

Working with the Moon involves listening rather than talking, and receiving rather than seeking or taking action to grasp at what we want. Clues about how we can do this are inherent to the nature of the celestial body. As mentioned, we can look to the waxing and waning of the moon to remind ourselves of life's creative ebb and flow and the continuous cycles of change that govern all life. Paying attention to the changing seasons of the Moon, and honoring these patterns, reminds us that times of withdrawal to reorient and ask the important questions about our path are a vital part of progress. These are the times to make adjustments and course corrections. Most importantly, this process can assist us in getting clear about the forces that drive us and what brings us the greatest fulfillment. Such clarity will keep the energy that has been stuck in the depths moving upward toward greater light and transcendence.

As the Moon traverses the night sky, it also shines its effusive light upon us as we dream. The realm of dreams is part of the great mystery of the human experience, next to death. It is the imaginal realm where we live out other lives—where we receive messages, process information, play out fears, resolve our confusion, and even, in some cases, receive communications from spirit guides or ancestors. Alejandro Jodorowsky once said, "The interpretation of dreams is a major part of the work of the artist-shaman-director-theater-clown-mystic in the search for that other form of madness, which is wisdom." In illuminating our dreams' messages, the Moon invites us to pay attention to these nighttime visions, for they provide clues to what emotional and soulful processes are taking place within us, and in doing so they show us what to focus on in our waking life.

And yes, working with psychedelics and plant medicines is another way to tap into the wisdom of our dreams and/or inner "visions" and awaken the symbolic aspects of the psyche to allow us to glean insight and make directional changes in our lives. Although not all psycho-active experiences involve visions, there is always a direct connection to the psyche, oftentimes cryptic or symbolic, but overflowing with emotional content and insight when reflected upon. We will talk more about dreams and their potential meaning further in the coming chapters. For now, let me show you how powerful it can be to channel the energy of the Moon to connect with guides or ancestors.

Making Peace with Jesus

I was invited to support a program for retired special forces, such as Navy Seals and other operations related teams, facilitating ibogaine sessions to aid with healing their PTSD and traumatic brain injury.

Several hours into the night the medicine had kicked in. One participant was tense and a bit irritated, and I could tell he was having a hard time.

As the night progressed, I sensed that he would benefit from connecting to his lunar side—something I had been specially trained to do in Bwiti, and that I'd helped others do many times. I asked him to imagine himself standing outside his home, then to look up at the sky and notice if it was day or night.

"Day," he responded.

"Change it to nighttime," I said in order to direct him to the lunar connection. I felt a bit of reluctance from him, but I sensed this lunar focus would help him relax and surrender to the difficulty he was experiencing and would help him understand how to engage with the medicine. I asked him to imagine in his mind's eye that he had thrust his fist up and was flying into the sky like Superman. "Keep flying past the clouds and into outer space, whizzing by the bright stars," I directed. "Now, stop and look behind you. What do you see?"

"I'm not really sure."

"Can you find Earth?" I asked. When he found Earth, I told him to look around and locate the Moon close by. "Once you've found it, fly to the Moon. Let me know when you've landed there."

Soon enough, his feet touched down on the Moon. We connected to the Moon by introducing ourselves in the following manner: full given name, mother's full maiden name, and father's full name. I asked the journeyer if there were any ancestors he would like to speak to. "No," he said bluntly. That is when I remembered that one of his intentions was to get right in his relationship with Jesus.

"Would you like to ask Jesus to visit?" I asked. He seemed open to the idea. So I said, "Then ask Jesus to come visit you on the Moon." Keep in mind that I usually would guide someone to call in a deceased relative; I had never thought of or even been asked to call in Jesus before. But I presumed that if he was a living man, he, too, was walking in the realms of the ancestors.

After the journeyer called Jesus in, there was a long pause. I asked him what was happening. Had Jesus shown up? "Yes," he stammered, "but he's not dressed in his normal clothes."

"Well, what is he wearing?"

"He's wearing a button-down shirt with slacks," he said, with a bit of a confused air.

"Oh, business-casual Jesus!" I chuckled. I sensed that Jesus had chosen an outfit that mirrored this man's typical wardrobe; perhaps he wanted to meet him on his level.

Next, I suggested he give Jesus a hug. "Tell him you love him," I added. He paused, and I sensed deep emotions stirring within him. After some time had passed, I gently continued, "Maybe see if Jesus will let you ask him some questions?" Once he got the green light from Jesus, I tuned in to what would help him with his reconnection to Christ, as he didn't have any questions prepared. It came to me. I said, "Ask Jesus, 'How can I make peace with you?'"

After another long pause, I asked him if Jesus had replied. His response will stay with me forever. Jesus told him: "I give love away, so you don't have to." This felt like exactly what the "real" Jesus would have said, as a figure representing unconditional love, and it seemed like what this man needed to hear to reconnect to him. The process felt complete.

This man struggled with grounding after his experience—not uncommon with iboga. I could sense the ruminations of his mind, as it tried to cast doubt on the realness of what had occurred. Afterward, I asked him about meeting Jesus, and his mood became less serious. He told me that when he'd hugged Jesus, it was a feeling like none other and probably the only time he'd felt "something" in the journey. "I can't really put words to the experience," he said, "but it felt like light and complete unconditional love that enveloped me."

"It sounds like you encountered the ineffable, something too great to be put into words," I said. He looked at me and smiled. I could see in his eyes that the concept had connected with him. He'd been all the way to the Moon, and he was softening.

Later, after he'd rested in a state of peace, he came to me and said, "I added a new word to my vocabulary: ineffable.*" It felt like his intention had manifested something mystical that planted seeds within his consciousness that strengthened his relationship with Jesus.*

· · · · · · · · · · · · · ·

SEEDING CONSCIOUSNESS IN PRACTICE

Moon Meditation

You, too, can repeat this same practice with the Moon in a meditation.

Travel to the Moon in your mind's eye, just like I described by imagining that you are flying there and landing on the Moon's crust. Once there, call in your ancestors or other archetypal figures whom you would like to connect with. First introduce yourself, like the journeyer above, by expressing your love for these figures. Then you can ask them a question or express something to them. Remember, there are no limits to what you can seek guidance on. They are in the spirit realm, so they can see everything. Listen deeply for what comes and notice any emotions or physical sensations accompanying the message. After you have finished speaking with them, thank them for connecting with you. Don't worry if you don't have any profound visions; not all people do. The purpose of this meditation is to tap into the energy of the Moon and connect to the wisdom of your ancestors. Use it as often as needed to give you strength and guidance. You can leave an offering for your ancestors, such as tobacco or something you know they loved, like a favorite food. You can also make an offering to the ancestors you did not know, in the form of fruit, nuts, or candy. It's best to leave this outside by a tree. This is how we make offerings in Bwiti. Trees may be spiritual antennas or conduits to reality's transcendent or non-material side. Now, pay attention, as these ancestors may continue to speak to you in dreams or through synchronicities in your waking life, or even through animal messengers such as birds or your pet. You can come back to this practice as often as you like.

Ancestral Wisdom

Ancient cultures place great value on the wisdom and experiences of their ancestors. This principle encourages learning from the past and honoring the legacy of those who came before us. Regardless of your relationship to your ancestral lineage, it is believed that our ancestors give us protection and strength, as spoken of from the Great Law of the Iroquois Confederacy and the practice of *Zheti-ata* in the Kazakhs clan of Mongol. Our previous seven generations of ancestors are standing behind us, and we are to take consideration of the next seven generations forward in our decision making.

Connecting intentionally with one's ancestors for support and wisdom is a timeless and universal practice that is present in a majority of ancient traditions. What specific wisdom might our ancestors hold? Just as our living elders can offer profound insights based on experiences accrued over a lifetime, our ancestral guides have knowledge garnered across the ages to impart. As such, they are especially gifted at providing messages that can support and comfort us in hard times, allowing us to place our trust in the greater cosmic unfolding and make difficult life decisions. The Moon is a bridge to this gift of connection.

And when we know how to listen, we also find that our ancestors communicate with us all the time, even if their messages come in subtle ways and sometimes take time to show up. You might hear them speaking to you through a song on the radio, through a child's imaginings, in the gaze of a pet's knowing eyes, or through the patterns of nature. The raven is known as a messenger from the ancestral realms—and I have woken up in the morning to ravens cawing at my door in times when I've reached out to my ancestors for support. Our ancestors often communicate with us through our dreams, sometimes simply by offering their presence. Psychedelics and plant medicines open the doorway for ancestors to make their presence known, sometimes through profoundly distinctive messages that give us goosebumps. The ancestors communicate their wisdom in the spaces of quiet and subtlety when we are paying attention in life. Therefore, it requires deep openness, listening, and presence to feel and connect with them.

To build a relationship to your ancestors, you can light a candle and make an altar to connect with them regularly. You might include photos of family members from previous generations, items that represent them, such as flowers they liked, or a keepsake that belonged to them. It is also important to note that even if we once had a difficult or abusive relationship with our ancestors, once they've returned to unseen realms they exist as their purest and most benevolent essence. Whatever misdeeds they may have committed in human form were a result of them operating from their egoic template and their own traumas. It may be hard to forgive these transgressions, but when we can connect to them as an ancestor, we open ourselves up to their guidance and support.

I recall one journey on a retreat where I worked, with a woman at who felt animosity toward her grandfather because of his substance abuse and overly masculine, domineering personality. In the session, her grandfather visited her, and she understood his pain for the first time;

she felt like she was processing it on behalf of her family. She could see how it had impacted her mother, who was judgmental about the idea of using psychedelics for healing, a worldview rooted in deep fear and a desire to protect her children from taking the same path as their great-grandfather, who had drowned his own pain with substances. The woman was able to release her shame along with the fears that emerged at the onset of entering an altered state, and she was ultimately able to surrender to the experience. Once she did, she felt a cosmic union that she described as blissful. She recalled feeling that she had become a woman for the first time, because she could feel her feminine power surging through her body, and she embraced it rather than trying to control or suppress it as she had in the past. This experience allowed her to feel compassion and forgiveness for her grandfather. His presence in her journey allowed for her feminine power to come through.

On a more macro level, studying how our ancient ancestors lived may offer valuable insights that counteract the dysfunction of modern life. For example, they did not have watches; they used the stars and nature to track time and map their coordinates within the cosmos. They understood that the position of certain stars in the sky contained information about when it was time to plant seeds and when it was time to rest. This wisdom alone reminds us that working against the cosmic order makes life more difficult. All things in nature exist within cycles of ripening, and once each stage of the cycle has passed, the time for action has expired.

For this reason, often when the ancients prayed, they did not ask for specific things; they asked instead whether it was the right time to do or have something. Working against time and out of sync with the natural cycles has been a hallmark of modern civilization, as it allows for the perpetual harvesting of resources—yet it creates immense suffering of humans and nature. This is the wisdom of the Moon. Doing what we can to work with these cycles, including our inner cycles, is an example of how we can apply ancestral wisdom in our daily lives.

The Portal

The equilibrium of our masculine and feminine energies, harmonized by the energies of the Sun and Moon, finds expression in the vesica piscis—a symbol composed of two intersecting circles, prevalent in ancient cultures and present in the iconic flower of life motif discovered in the Osirian temple in Abydos. Representing fertility and the genesis of new life in its myriad forms, the vesica most likely inspired the Venn diagram. The place of intersection in the middle represents the divine marriage of spirit and matter, called *hieros gamos* by the ancient Greeks. That convergence point, often referred to as "the portal," is believed to serve as a gateway to the higher mystical dimensions.

By balancing Sun and Moon, we also allow the right and left hemispheres of the brain to align, crucial for bringing forth ingenuity, as seeded by the insights gained from traversing the innerverse. In the human brain, the portal is represented by the corpus callosum, a large bundle of more than 200 million myelinated nerve fibers that connect the two brain hemispheres, permitting communication between the right and left sides of the brain. A recent 2022 research study by Simonsson et al. titled "Preliminary Evidence of Links Between Ayahuasca Use and the Corpus Callosum" demonstrates that ritual users of the psychoactive brew ayahuasca possess a thicker neuronal density of the corpus callosum (2022). Those who can master both the sciences (left brain, masculine) and the arts (right brain, feminine) tend to have a more well-developed corpus callosum. According to a study on Albert Einstein's brain, by Weiwei Men et al. Florida State University in 2014, shows his left and right hemispheres were remarkably well connected, a factor that may have contributed to his genius. As Tom Cowan, mystic and author, articulated, "Mystical insight and enlightenment occur when the veil between the worlds is lifted, the worlds are bridged, the gap closes, and we cross over."

By bridging force and receptivity, action and stillness, power, and humility, we create a portal to the sacred—that great creative force that animates all life. By honoring both the Sun and Moon, fire and water, Mother and Father, yin and yang, Dark and Light, movement and stillness, we begin to experience the world not as a place of competition and polarity but as a place of nonduality and, within this, endless potential. Here you may see a similarity to the alchemical process, but in this case we're moving from a place of integrating both the inner and outer worlds. To do this, we must learn to temper our egoic urges to push forward no matter what and instead learn to find comfort in stillness. This requires us to befriend our shadow parts—for they await us in the dark—and look to them as the teachers that they are. The Moon is essential in seeding consciousness as it is the doorway through which we enter the murky waters of our psyche. High-dose or mystical-experience inducing plant medicine and psychedelic initiations can provide in depth work. Still, it is also possible to balance Sun and Moon energies in everyday life by aligning our actions with the phases of the lunar cycle—from new, waxing, full, and waning, and into the midnight of the dark moon. Most importantly, we achieve this balance through regular check-ins with the Moon within.

All creative projects, all healing processes, and all relationships follow the universal patterns of inception, birth, completion, death, and rebirth, as displayed by the Moon on her nightly traverse of the night sky. These phases speak to the continual work of bringing the denser aspects of our psyche into the light, to be transmuted and released through inner alchemy. The seeds are planted right at the beginning of this process, when the light of the Moon is almost entirely hidden, right before the new moon initiates the next creation cycle. For this reason, the night before each new moon can be a powerful moment to go within and ask what is ready to be seeded and birthed next in our lives.

Reflecting on your connection to these phases, can you recall when you were creating something and things just weren't flowing? Maybe you had brain fog or simply felt blocked. Could it be possible that you started at a less supportive time? Perhaps the energies you attempted to tap into were not there to nurture your process. As frustrating as it can be to have to wait until the timing is right, our culture of urgency has arisen from our over-reliance on solar modes of living. We can sometimes keep pushing against or out of sync with the lunar cycles, only to end up even more frustrated after spending an entire day on a project and feeling we haven't created anything, or that we'll have to redo our work.

Again, this illustrates how counterproductive it is to press forward regardless, forgetting that taking time to step back, rest, and assess is equally important. Working against the forces of nature just creates suffering, strife, and burnout. All things in nature have their own cycles. What is yours? There is a gift that unfolds in the mystery as we honor each phase of the creative process to efficiently draw forth material from the more feminine or maternal forces, to harness the ethers of our imagination. This is what the Moon wants to teach us: to be masterful artists.

Ultimately, our connection to Aluna helps us tap into our creative excellence and, in doing so, take our place as co-creators within the greater web of life. It is part of our work to actively develop a relationship with our lunar side.

As mentioned earlier in the book, I don't want you to follow any of the instructions presented here like a cookbook recipe, or to try to "brainify" this process. I want to encourage you to show up with intention and to simply feel, as you engage in the work of connecting with your inner moon. Feel that natural Moon algorithm in your body like the beat to your favorite song, and dance with it. As with divinity itself, your relationship with the Moon is *your* relationship with the Moon. It is unique to you and the Moon. This might look different for everybody. One person I met had talked to the Moon via a screen that appeared in his mind's eye, with words that looked like they were being typed. Others might feel the whisper of an emotion that contains all the lunar wisdom they need at that moment. You might not experience or feel anything at all. Don't be disappointed. Just keep cultivating that connection.

The moon that metaphorically lives inside you and the one hanging in the night sky are interconnected as your teachers. Both are there to support you as you build your connection to the Moon and learn to honor her quiet, shadowy ways. Since she is the keeper of the psychic realms, she can respond to the questions to which you thought you would never find answers.

. . . .

SEEDING CONSCIOUSNESS IN PRACTICE
Lunation Reflections

This meditation helps you connect with the Moon, enhance your intuition, and embrace the cyclic nature of life.

Start by finding a quiet and comfortable space, seated in a chair or on the floor. Close your eyes and take a few deep breaths. Breathe in and out through your nose to calm and balance your nervous system. Set an intention for how you would like to connect to the Moon.

See the Moon in your mind's eye, glowing in the dark night sky. Focus on its shape, size, and color. Let the moonlight wash over you, flowing through the top of your head and into your body. Feel the feminine, watery beams illuminating your entire body.

Now see the Moon transitioning into its phases. Begin with the new moon, and gradually watch it progress through the waxing crescent, first quarter, waxing gibbous, full moon, waning gibbous, third quarter, and finally the waning crescent phase. As you visualize each phase, feel the energy within you ebb and flow.

With each moon cycle, allow yourself to be more in tune with your inner wisdom and intuition. Take note of any insights or messages that arise and welcome any guidance from the Moon.

Once you are complete with connecting with each cycle, return your focus to your breath. Feel your feet and hands, and slowly open your eyes. Take a moment to reflect. Write down anything you felt or received during this meditation.

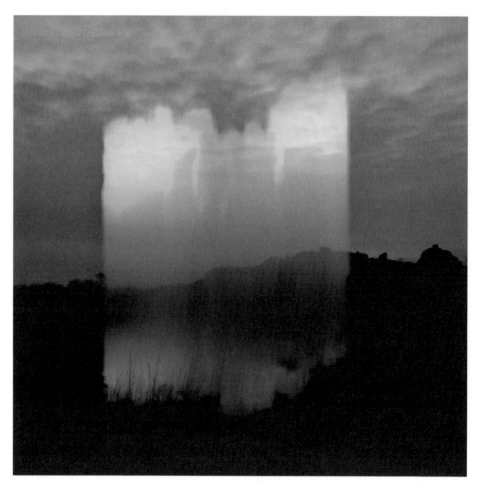

Mesquite Imprint

by Lela Amparo

9

Tuning In

Becoming a Receiver of Consciousness

*Intuition becomes increasingly valuable in the new
information society precisely because there is so much data.*

JOHN NAISBITT

Ultimately the ailment plaguing the Western world, spurring interest in
plant medicines and psychedelics, underscores our profound estrange-
ment from intuition—the innate, instinctual connection to the spirit
world and our true essence. Rediscovering our innate intuitive faculties
is crucial; it is to the benefit of all beings and the planet herself as it will
give essential instructions to move forward. The more we can tune back
in, the more our sensitivity and receptivity will return to us, and the more
aligned our actions and lives will be with the great web of life. This journey demands the practice of introspection and receiving guidance, rooting out the weeds hindering the flourishing of intuition within us.

As we have learned, the body is a cosmic intelligence receiver.
Through our bodies and by tuning in to our inner moon, or subconscious, we reunite our innerverse with the entire universe. When this
connection is established and strong, we experience an abundance of
well-being and synchronicity in our lives. The more connected we are,
the less resistance we will face in the form of fear or other blocks. Not

that fear doesn't show up at all, but the more we find ourselves living in a natural state of flow and receptivity, the more we see that we are always protected and have access to what we need. This results in a high level of coherence with the natural order, greater emotional stability, lowered stress levels, and increased mental clarity.

Tuning in to our inner moon and asking for assistance from the spirit world, as I have guided you in the previous two chapters, is the albedo part of inner alchemy. Psychedelics can aid us greatly in this, as they help us tap into the information transmitted throughout the greater web. The tools in this chapter will take us a step deeper into this ability to receive guidance with or without psychedelics. A spider weaves a perfect web; as a gap in the arachnid's design could mean a missed meal opportunity, we need to intentionally plug into the web of life so we can receive life-supporting insights. Our ability to listen in and to divine the information necessary to support us depends on the extent to which we can see beyond the interference we encounter in our daily lives, much of which is generated by the chattering of the ego. This will clear your channel and guide you on your own path in building this connection.

Our job, then, is to gather and assimilate this information and eventually move into right action as we apply our knowledge to the choices we're tasked with making in our lives, choices that impact us as individuals and have a ripple effect on the broader world. This last part is the rubedo phase of inner alchemy, which we will discuss in depth in chapter 10. For now, I want to show you how to decipher the intuitive hits, sensory knowing, metaphysical dream states, and psychedelic visions that live in the realm of Aluna and contain vital information with which to seed our consciousness.

Becoming a Receiver

Psychedelic and plant medicine journeys are an access point to the symbolic mind, the place of visions, intuition, and numinous insights.

Although not all information in our journeys can be usefully translated and often is far from literal, many of the tools for dream interpretation can be applied to psychedelic visionary content. Journeyers sometimes experience hallucinations when their eyes are closed but can equally encounter a distorted reality with their eyes wide open. This is due to the activation of specific receptors in the brain, primarily serotonin transporters, which opens us up to transmissions occurring outside of regular human perception. This hyper-awareness enables us to "zoom in" like a microscope, allowing for profoundly deep insights.

We are constantly receiving information in our daily lives. But the more intently we listen, and the more we can dial down the volume on the noise of the outside world and our own thoughts, the more access we have to the subtle nuances of the messages that are being communicated. As a medicine woman, sometimes I act as an intermediary, receiving and interpreting messages on my journeyer's behalf, when appropriate, and carefully do so as to empower the querant to tune in themselves. My ability to connect to the spirit world and tune in to channels of subtle information allows me to collect wisdom to support the individuals I work with. I do my best not to color it with my own lenses of perception but instead gently offer something that might have meaning to the person, either in the moment or later on. And while some of us can access this connection more easily than others, we all have the capacity. Our intuitive connection to the great web of life is an innate gift that grants us true inner power and sovereignty—and tuning in is what gives us greater sanction to follow our unique destiny and find our purpose. This access to life's web cannot be taken away; no matter how strong or weak one's connection is, it can always be refined and cultivated. We must be humble and realize that symbolic interpretation is more of an art than a science. I have seen, time and again, that as we return to our true selves, our innate intuitive abilities naturally awaken and become enhanced. Psychedelics and plant medicines can act as bridges that open us to insights and can support a deeper connection to our intuitive capacity.

As I've discussed, the first step in strengthening our intuition is to seek balance: rather than succumbing to overreliance on the solar mode of being that is always chasing or seeking, we must shift toward a receptive orientation of learning to simply be and receive. This means letting go of any specific goal or desired result in our journeywork and allowing whatever wants to come, to come. Something beyond what you ever imagined may show up, opening the door to untold possibilities. That is the beauty of this work. There is an art to letting things come to you. It requires patience and discipline. But it always begins by simply showing up—in ceremony with psychedelics or other plant medicines, perhaps—and then listening for clues. If nothing comes, then rather than going looking, we can ask to be shown what we need to see, as we keep "listening" with all our senses. A previously hidden "doorway" almost always appears; we must be brave and curious enough to walk through it.

How do we know this is the right path of inner inquiry for us? A simple mantra to follow is: *Wait to be invited.* Personally, when I am being called forward, I get a "yes" feeling that causes shivers in my body; in the same way, I might experience nauseating anxiety in my stomach when something is a "no." This may be different for you. Try asking yourself and feeling what your "yes" and "no" are. It takes practice, but once you feel it, it becomes one of your most valuable intuitive tools.

When we actively push forward without getting the proper signals or by assigning meaning that may not be accurate to signals, we are more likely to find ourselves traveling down the wrong path—and perhaps even landing on our faces. By instead practicing *allowing* we can trust that what naturally comes our way is ours to receive. In addition, allowing is a remedy for imposter syndrome: when something is meant for us, it always shows up at exactly the right time, whether or not we feel "ready" for it. Sometimes intuitive clues can show us something very far in the future that we're being prepared for but aren't yet ready to receive. The best practice is to keep following the trail of breadcrumbs and letting go of what we think we know.

So how do we tune in? Developing an acute sensitivity to our feelings is a necessary prerequisite for receiving and interpreting symbolic messages. We do this by practicing balancing our solar and lunar energies and replacing "doing" with "being" whenever we can. As discussed, our ability to sense these subtle inner cues is often hindered by living a hectic, fast-paced lifestyle and by the chaotic noise of the outside world. The discomfort or disharmony this creates urges us to seek answers outside ourselves rather than going within. But suppose we are always exerting our energy outwardly. In that case, we are left with very little bandwidth for tuning in to our inner wisdom and receiving intelligent feedback designed to help return *us* to the center of our lives.

Our feelings—communicated through both emotional and sensory feeling states—are the key to divination, which is the art of interpreting messages from the unseen realms. In numerous traditions worldwide, both past and present, there are many techniques for interpreting the omens and auguries of the unseen world. For example, this practice can be done using cowrie shells, tea leaves, tree bark, bones, tarot cards, runes, or coins. The Kogi Kággaba mamos read the movement of bubbles from water to divine the future. These tools help the diviner communicate with ancestors, utilize the elements, and explore immaterial reality. Some divination practices, such as dowsing or using a pendulum, give simple "yes" or "no" answers—often in a "felt sense" in the body. Such techniques can be sources of knowledge to test or validate your intuitive senses regarding binary yes/no decisions in life.

This is where psychedelics help us again: they are connectors. They bridge the seen and unseen realms between body, mind, and soul. For example, they may connect us with ancestors who have passed to the other side, with feelings of grief that have been stuffed away for many years, or with information about your life's true purpose that has been hidden by doubts or limiting self-beliefs. The more clearly we can see a message, the easier it becomes to divine its meaning and act on what we are being shown, as we shake off the limitations of the egoic template and begin to live our destinies.

Sometimes the spirit world communicates in the most magical but symbolic ways. I remember once in a journeywork session with a woman, the answer to a question she asked was shown to be a painting by renowned graffiti artist Banksy, depicting a little girl reaching toward a red heart-shaped balloon that has just escaped her grasp. I asked this woman what it represented. As an avid art collector, she felt it spoke to surrender and release of attachment. This piece of art has a significant story behind it: It went up for auction at Sotheby's, reaching a record $25.4 million at the closing of bidding. Spectators watched with gaping jaws as the painting started to move, slowly shredding itself, as if the artist had put some self-destruct mode in place. The shredding process stopped about two-thirds of the way through—a malfunction of the artist's stunt, many speculate. As I tap into the complexity that this piece represented on so many levels, I think of the Japanese concept of *wabi sabi*, the beauty of imperfection and impermanence.

One day after this, I was on the beach, and in the sky, an object sparkling in the distance caught my eye. I watched it fly down from the heavens and land in the ocean. It was the red heart balloon that the girl from the Banksy piece had lost. I rescued it from the ocean shore. Now this story had touched me. The beauty of its message lies in showing the value of the bigger picture, rather than attachment to particular things. This relates back to the mindset one must have in order to access their intuition.

I have attended some workshops to learn about a martial art called Merpati Putih, which comes from Indonesia. The name translates to "white dove." The claim of this lineage, which was passed down royal bloodlines, is that intuition is a skill to be cultivated and developed. There are masters of the tradition who can drive a car blindfolded, just using their intuition, or what might be referred to in some Eastern traditions as the "third eye." In my first Merpati Putih workshop, after doing practices involving breathwork and meditation, I wore a blindfold and navigated through an obstacle course, using my intuition to see. Although I will not teach you this specific practice, I will share some basic tools that can help you tap into your power to use and direct your intuition.

Presence

Before we discuss the art of divination in more depth, it is important to create the right conditions for tuning. The more we can ground ourselves, staying physically and energetically present, the deeper the quality and nuance of the information we receive becomes, and the more we can trust it. I often see people picking apart their visions while the medicine is still in conversation with them, trying to make sense of something too soon. When the mind rushes to do this, it impedes the process of receiving. Oftentimes an initial revelation is just a sneak preview for a grander tapestry of realization or connection. Practicing presence teaches us to be patient and to wait for the fullness of the message to be revealed—which may occur weeks or months after a psychedelic journey.

This is why meditation is a key practice in many wisdom traditions and centrally relevant to working with psychedelics. Meditation allows us to observe, detach from our thoughts, and sink more deeply into presence. This, in turn, helps us develop a sense of non-attachment. Non-attachment means not giving any particular desire or outcome your attention. It allows you to truly surrender to what is, and to take a more curious approach to life. The objective is for the individual to become an empty vessel, a neutral recipient of consciousness.

When interviewing someone interested in working with psychedelics and plant medicines, I ask if they practice meditation regularly. If so, I ask how long they have been practicing, which helps me gauge their comfort level with non-doing introspection and meta-awareness. This is important because psychoactive plants amplify thoughts and cognitive patterns. Suppose someone has had the experience of sitting quietly, learning how to focus their attention, and not reacting to whatever arises in the moment. If they've already learned to do this, they're usually better able to manage it even in an altered state of consciousness.

Those with untrained minds can at times become overwhelmed, reactive, or over-identified with their amplified, racing thoughts, emotions, and internal noise. Many suffer in altered states of consciousness because of this—which can limit how far one progresses in the depth of work. Conversely, the internal spaciousness and centeredness created through a regular meditation practice can unlock the immense potential of psychedelics and plant medicines and the altered states they induce.

Clearing the Space

Your environmental space may be occupied with unwanted guests that are invisible to the naked eye, such as spirits, old or stagnant forces, and residual emotions. The practice of ritualistic cleansing uses medicinal plants or resins to purify and protect a space, person, or object before ceremonial work, by using burning to intentionally produce smoke. This practice can dispel negative energies, promote spiritual and emotional healing, and create a harmonious atmosphere. It is a fundamental protocol in most wisdom traditions, as it helps dissipate forces that may conflict with our ability to receive information clearly from the spirit world. Often, an individual's emotional disturbances during a psychedelic initiation are linked to being in spaces where the energy needs to be cleared. Traditional ceremonialists burn sacred aromatic plants and resins like sage, tobacco, frankincense, myrrh, copal, palo santo, yerba santa, oud, dragon's blood, sweetgrass, cedar, and incense to clear energies in an environment and welcome positive spirits. In my tradition, Bwiti, we use a sacred resin torch from the okoume tree to clear the space, communicate with the spirit world, and cleanse negative energies from individuals. We also perform a ritual smoke bath called *effulu*, for which a smoke tent is created where an individual can be fully enveloped—a means of purification during initiation.

Research shows that sage has antibacterial properties and eliminates harmful airborne microbes from the air. Additional studies suggest that smudging rituals encourage increased focus and attention, which supports the idea that these plants assist the act of prayer and intentional thoughts. The smell of burned sage is also proven to help improve sleep and reduce anxiety. But it is important to know that this ancient practice's popularity increases demand for plants and resins like sage, copal, oud, and palo santo, which are now over-harvested. Steer away from wild-harvested sage, as its use may threaten the species' survival, and many native peoples have asked that Westerners seek alternatives. Look for sustainably farmed sage or cultivate your own sage plant at home. Also, consider burning lavender, rosemary, or mugwort, which are sustainable alternatives.

Ceremonial cleansing, meanwhile, is taken very seriously and incorporates many involved rituals, including personal purification protocols. In the Mēxica tradition, the women carrying the *copalero* or *popoxcomitl*, the copal resin burner, go into a special forty- to fifty-two-day process to consecrate the copalero. This involves rituals performed around the moon cycles, introducing the copalero to each of the four elements, and abstaining from sex throughout the process. If the copalero is broken or cracked, it is buried, and the process must be done over. I share this to emphasize how seriously this practice is taken—and that it's valuable to exercise this level of intentionality in cleansing your space before attempting to tune in.

The best way for you to practice cleansing is to use intention and remember to be thorough. You can use prayer and clearly state the area you intend to clear, and call upon support in your process through prayer. Vaporizing sustainably harvested essential oils is another subtle but effective way of clearing the space.

188 ⊙ Tuning In

Opening the Channel

In addition to cleansing our ceremonial spaces, the body—our primary "tool" for divination—should be clear internally before we tune in. One tribe of the Peruvian Amazon, the Shipibo, observe a special diet that is designed to elevate their sensitivities to better "hear" the subtle energies of the natural world. These diets, or *dietas*, allow Shipibo ancestral healers to communicate with plants and animals and even diagnose and treat illnesses. A dieta can last anywhere from two weeks to several months, a year, or even longer, and generally requires eliminating any salt, fats, fermented foods, sugar, red meat, dairy, spices, fried foods, alcohol, caffeine, or pharmaceutical drugs. Many dietas also forbid using media, reading books, engaging in sexual intercourse or sensuous activity, and using personal care products with synthetic ingredients or perfumes. The dietary requirements are put in place because these things are thought to stir up "noise" or interference inside us, which prevents us from truly hearing with our spiritual senses.

Fasting is another way we can open our listening channels and is a spiritual technology observed by traditional communities across the world, from early Gnostics to modern-day Indigenous peoples of the Americas. The view is that food, especially meat, weighs the body down, preventing subtle receptivity, digestion diverts the energies required for our mystical faculties to operate, and stepping away from desire is a sacrifice we make as an offering for the opening of communication it provides. The Mēxica peoples, believed to be the descendants of the famous Aztec Empire in Mexico, observe a rite of passage known as a vision quest. The vision quest typically involves an initiate abstaining from food and water for several days while sitting in isolation somewhere in the wilderness. Vision quests also form part of many North American Indigenous rites of passage. In this case, the combination of fasting from both food and outside stimuli often brings about a mystical visionary experience induced by the stresses of an extreme environment, deprivation, and being forced to face one's deepest fears.

These fasts are usually accompanied by sacred fires that burn to protect participants, and songs that deliver them strength or spiritual sustenance from the ancestral world. The Mēxica and other traditions around the world also enact sacred rituals and prayers to protect the fasting individuals. Intense fasts such as these should never be done without proper guidance and support.

For most of us, consuming light meals consisting of pure, organic food is ideal for supporting our spiritual work. On my past retreats, I design a menu consisting of mostly plant-based recipes; I avoid soy, gluten, and inflammatory foods such as non-sprouted beans, nuts, and nightshades like tomatoes and peppers. All meals are cooked with coconut or olive oil, since oils made from ingredients like safflower, corn, and rice bran are also inflammatory, causing a response in the body that diverts psychic energy or creates unnecessary internal noise that dulls one's capacity to tune in.

The Inner Eye

Once the channels have been opened by getting present, clearing the space, and preparing the physical body to receive information, we have the proper setting to begin the tuning in process. When you sit down to play an instrument, you want to ensure it is tuned properly before you start making music. In this case, the "music" is in the visions and other transmissions we receive through our senses.

On a purely physiological level, visionary experiences can be interpreted and identified as electrical or chemical activity in the brain. Yet these visionary states additionally serve an esoteric, invisible, and unquantifiable function, with symbolic meaning and communication from our subconscious mind. Scientists tend to approach the phenomenology of dreams from a reductionist perspective, attributing visions we receive during dream states to random electrochemical firing and hormonal activity. These visions are often dismissed as mere psychological projections or the byproducts of biological processes. Such overly rational and materialist explanations minimize the transcendent, archetypal, and spiritual nature of what mystics and saints have perceived and encountered for millennia, pointing to what ultimately lies beyond our limited waking, three-dimensional perception. In my experience, our dreams and other hallucinatory visions are often allegorical symbols transmitted from the spirit world.

The antenna through which we receive these visions is the *epiphysis cerebri*, also known as the pineal gland, as found in the brains of most vertebrates. The role of this endocrine gland is commonly understood as regulating sleep and dream cycles. The pineal gland produces melatonin, serotonin, 5-MeO-DMT, N,N-DMT, and pinoline. The fact that our bodies naturally produce these "psychedelic" molecules shows that humans are designed to experience the states they bring about, and that psychedelic inner visions are an important and natural part of the human experience. Meanwhile the outer layer of this chamber-like gland is made of calcite microcrystals; ancient Taoists called this gland the "crystal palace." Just as Mantak Chia explains in his book *Darkness Technology*, this place is an alchemist's kitchen where calcium crystals vibrate, releasing melatonin that then goes through a metamorphic conversion into serotonin, 5-MeO-DMT, N,N-DMT, and pinoline. All endogenous tryptamines go through creation and transformation in this crystal palace. Just like the original limestone outer casing of the Great Pyramid of Giza, the vibration of the crystals in the temple of our brains also generates a piezoelectric current that produces a voltage from pressure or heat. The ancients were aware that this creates a field around the body, turning it into a transistor radio that sends and receives signals. Hieroglyphs and artwork found in ancient Egyptian temples contain information that continues to intrigue researchers around this topic, offering insights into ancient wisdom that is not yet fully understood by modern scholarship.

In the context of spiritual practices, such as those related to seeding consciousness, this piezoelectric energy may enhance our ability to access deeper states of consciousness, intuition, and spiritual insight. By understanding and harnessing this natural energy within our brains, we may be able to facilitate communication with higher realms, ancestors, and spiritual beings, leading to personal transformation, healing, and spiritual growth. Although research is limited, "The Role of Piezoelectricity in Meditation and Spiritual Practices" by J. J. Hurtak and Desiree Hurtak, published in the *Journal of Spirituality and Consciousness Studies*, explores this topic. Another peer-reviewed research paper, "Piezoelectricity and the Spiritual Body: Exploring the Mysteries of Energy and Consciousness," is available in the *International Journal of Transpersonal Studies*.

The Vedic traditions also recognize the pineal gland as the third eye, which governs our intuition or "sixth sense." This further supports the evidence that the pineal gland functions as the intermediator for messages transmitted from the subconscious, the spirit world, and the intuitive domains. The key lies in unlocking these inner gateways to receive insights guiding us toward answers or direction.

Guidance for Inquiry

Language is the first thing that comes to mind when we think of "inquiry." But requesting information and interpreting the inner visions we've received—either during a psychedelic initiation or through other intentional dream states—is a process that often goes beyond words and requires us to expand our definition of "language." In essence, language consists of vibration, sound, and current. But any sound frequency carries an intelligence and an intention beyond the spoken word. As Indigenous methodologies expert Lila Liberman describes, "That which appears as tangible is a hallucinatory living veil between octaves of understanding and perception, with the midwife of language in between." In each moment, the whole universe is communicating with us through a language of symbols and feeling states. Every atom is vibrating in relationship to and in conversation with life; with every exhale, something else responds to or receives the energy being released.

Another way to think about this is that we use language to create both stories and spells. The stories we tell ourselves and others are often a way of interpreting feelings or emotions that arise from our personal experiences. What happens when we examine a traumatic event through a different lens and tell a different story? How do our stories color our lives and emit vibrations that influence what comes back to us? We are weaving reality with every word we say, and with the feelings or intentions behind our words. This is especially important to remember when we are tuning in, asking for answers from the spirit world.

To avoid interpreting messages through the lens of our egoic template, the seat of all the desires and aversions built to "protect" us, it is important to remain neutral in our queries to the spirit world. As an exercise, I write out my questions before I tune in to my own internal guidance—whether under the influence of psychedelics or not. I then run my questions by other trusted intuitive guides, or I use divination tools such as tarot cards to check that my questions are not colored with my own underlying beliefs or desires for specific outcomes. Some examples of ways in which I may open a question are as follows:

Is it advisable at this time to . . . ?

What steps must I take to accomplish . . . ?

What kind of approach would be supportive in accomplishing . . . ?

Is it in my highest alignment to have . . . ?

What obstacles must I clear in relation to . . . ?

Does it serve my highest purpose to . . . ?

These questions contain neutrality because they focus on timing, process, support, obstacles, and alignment rather than specific outcomes or clear-cut instructions on what I should or shouldn't do. They acknowledge that pathways are opening, and timelines are shifting every moment, leaving plenty of space for the unknowable to show up.

No matter what our intention or question is, it is tough for this not to be colored by an underlying desire or belief. Profound clarification comes with writing questions in a journal while reworking them several times, which can help you more clearly communicate your needs to the spirit world. We should also use positive language when communicating with spirits and be careful not to use profanity, cursing, or a negative tone that shows disrespect.

Instead, use expansive language that flows from your heart and that is designed to help you receive insight from outside your current perception of a given situation. You could ask yourself, "How might my feelings around this situation be clouding my insight?" This will ensure you don't limit what information you can receive, and that you let go of all expectations. For example, compare how you feel when you ask, "How can I prevent my heart from being broken?" with "How may I step into having a deeper sense of self-love and strength?" In this instance, if your query is colored by an underlying belief that people are out to break your heart, then you will keep manifesting that pattern in your life as a self-fulfilling prophecy.

Before invoking your query, you can also take a moment to imagine receiving the exact answers you need. How does it feel to "know" you are on the right path? Breathe into that feeling. Anchor it in your body by fully experiencing the feeling. For instance, if you are calling money or a new home for yourself, feel the emotions of peace and support that you would have if it came flowing in. This is not about "manifestation" but about inviting your body and nervous system to allow for the possibility. Staying open to possibilities allows us to receive information fully and for the great mystery of life to surprise us. A study headed by the Swiss Federal Institute of Sport in 2016 demonstrated that visualization helps athletes improve their performance, but what if these same athletes used intuitive practices throughout the process to understand what they were facing, and asked what would be the most effective way to prepare? I sense that athletic performance levels would reach another benchmark of excellence. I encourage you to try the ideas above before embarking on a psychedelic or plant medicine journey. If you're open to making inquiries, then you can start to receive guidance, which may help you prepare for situations you encounter in life.

These methods help me to get clear when I am unsure about something. They also allow me to develop further questions and reflections that I may not yet have considered. More often than not, they present new information that hasn't occurred to me. Often a situation may call for several angles of questioning before I can obtain a full picture. This practice has, over time, supported me in cultivating non-attachment when receiving information—preventing my egoic distortions from interfering with or misinterpreting the messages I receive.

Dreamwork and Visionary Interpretation

The dream or visionary space is a channel to receive the rich and diverse seeds of potential germinating within ourselves. Perhaps the dream space is the "seed bank" of cosmic potential. The visionary phenomenology that arises in plant medicine and psychedelic journeys occasionally can be so vivid and rapid that you can barely track what you're seeing or make sense of it. Don't worry; it will return if it's important and relevant. This part of the chapter will provide some sense-making tools that can help you integrate the experience's visionary aspects. Although you don't have to embark on a psychedelic journey or deliberately access altered states of consciousness to receive powerful and profound inner visions; we all do this naturally when we dream, whether we can remember our dreams or not. Dreamwork is one way to begin accessing cosmic intelligence every day—or at night. In addition, either the spirit of the medicine or an individual's ancestors will often start communicating with them through the dream state in the lead-up to any ceremony or initiation.

Both visionary psychedelic experiences and dreams are important communication mediums for the psyche and spirit world. The Aboriginal rites of passage, such as walkabouts in the Australian territories, or vision quests among the Original Peoples of Northern and Central America, use practices to induce visions that often shape the entirety of one's life. Our visions support us in receiving answers, which, in turn, help to remove psychic blockages as we gain insightful new perspectives that may have been obscured from us in our waking reality. But the subconscious sometimes has nonsensical ways of relaying information. Interpreting the messages one receives from their psyche or inner guides sometimes feels like trying to decipher the meaning of a surrealist work of art, or playing Pictionary with a four-year-old. Although visions can sometimes be straightforward, they are rarely meant to be taken literally but, more often, to evoke deeper insights and contemplation.

When I was in South Africa supporting the creation of the Declaration for the Protection of Sacred Sites by the Alliance for the Sacred Sites of Earth Gaia (ASSEGAIA), we engaged in a dreamwork session to get guidance from the ancestors, led by several *sangomas*, traditional healers in South Africa. Ceremonial dreamwork is one way to use dreams as a communication tool in the unseen world. Ceremonial fire often inaugurates the dreamwork, and grass mats or blankets are placed on the earth around the fire for the group to lie on, before prayers and intentions are expressed to open up the space for listening to the ancestors and guiding spirits. The group gathers around the fire for protection as they rest. Throughout the night, visions come through to those open to receiving them. The next morning, dreams are shared amongst the group, while usually one or several oracles or seers are present to help individuals interpret the meanings of these messages. These types of dreaming rituals can be meant for individual guidance, for teaching younger adepts, or supporting the broader village or tribe. The Kogi Kággaba engage in a similar ritual of constructing ceremonial houses of original thought for the purpose of this important work.

As with our own inner visions, our psyche speaks to us through symbols in dreams. These scenes only sometimes make sense or carry the continuity of a linear storyline. However, each "actor" in the dream always represents a part of you or a feeling or attitude toward a situation—a guiding concept that can be applied both to our regular dreams and to visionary psychedelic phenomena of a surrealistic nature.

Here are a couple of examples dream interpretations:

The dreamer has an eagle as a pet and ventures down into a cave that is identified as a mine.

In this dream, the eagle could represent the dreamer's power. The mine might represent them preparing for deep inner excavation. In this case, I recognized the symbology of this dream from my years of practice working with dreams and visionary states. Still, it can often be necessary to look deeper into what the symbols represent and what they mean to the individual. For instance, let's say the person has a passion for falconry, and they have a falcon land on their arm in a dream. The falcon could represent them pursuing their passions or hobbies. Maybe they are taking life too seriously, and the message is that they need to prioritize activities that feed their soul.

The dreamer sees his teacher naked in a bathtub while talking to him.

In this case, the teacher in the bath could represent the theme of purification. The fact that the dreamer is talking to the teacher in the bath also represents the teacher's vulnerability. The dream could show the dreamer that he will learn a lesson from the teacher about how to work with vulnerability.

Perhaps more important than the dream, vision, or hallucination itself is the underlying emotional tone of the content. Symbolic information is rarely literal in meaning and is nearly always allegorical in nature. Some fundamental questions to ask in a dream or visionary interpretation are:

What does that person or image represent to you?

What emotions did you feel?

What was the mood of the dream or vision like?

It is easy to run a search on the internet or look in a dream book for the "spiritual" or "symbolic" meaning of specific animals, aspects, and archetypes within a dream. But what's more important is what that thing means to you, and how it makes you feel.*

You can also use the dream space to connect to the ancestors or the spirit world. If you have a specific question, remember to introduce yourself to the spirit world by saying your full name, your mother's full (maiden) name, and your father's full name when you get into bed at night. Then, if you know it, call in the full name of the ancestor you want to connect with. Ask them your question and thank them for their help. First thing when you wake up, take a notebook and write down anything you remember from your dreams that night. Often the meaning will become clear in the form of an intuitive hit as you commit your recollections to paper.

---

*However, some ancient texts that help interpret the symbolism found in dreams are Artemidorus's *The Interpretation of Dreams*, Aristotle's *On Divination in Sleep*, and Hippocrates's *Regimen 4*.

Dream and visionary symbolism play out in our waking reality too. But to see it, we must learn to slow down, connect to our inner moon, and become the observer of our lives. As Carl Jung stated, "Salvation is a long road that leads through many gates. These gates are symbols. Each new gate is at first invisible; it seems it must be created, for it exists only if one has dug up the spring's root, the symbol."

Every situation we experience has deep symbolic meaning for us. It is always a reflection of our psyche and the greater cosmic order of which we are inextricably a part. Tuning in to the trail of breadcrumbs our soul has left for us, using whatever tools we have access to, maps the forward route that is beckoning to our primordial intelligence. When we pay close enough attention, this trail reveals itself without us having to look for it. Our waking experience is a perpetual unfolding of the seen and unseen forces at play, which dynamically coalesce in the material world that surrounds us. The path is there in the small synchronicities that feel like a nod from the universe, such as repeating numbers on a clock, or a word spelled out by the license plate on a car.

Again, ask yourself: What does this mean for me? What could my ancestors and spirit guides be attempting to communicate? You will know your divination skills are on point when this is accompanied by an "aha!" moment or a jolt that might even make the hairs on your arms stand on end, bringing you into a deeper understanding of yourself or a situation. As James Grotstein, professor of psychology at UCLA, asks, "Who is the dreamer who dreams the dream?" This question allows the seeds of awareness and insight surging through the web of life to be planted in our consciousness, where they can help us blossom and grow.

. . . .

SEEDING CONSCIOUSNESS IN PRACTICE
Tuning In

Choose a time of day when you are not hungry but feel relatively empty. Find a quiet and comfortable space to sit or lie down in,

without distractions. Have a journal or notepad close by to write notes
or insights.

Begin by ceremonially cleansing the space with the smoke of aromatic plants and resins like frankincense, copal, or palo santo. Find a comfortable position and deepen your breath, focusing on slowly feeling the sensations of the breath leaving and entering your nose. Set an intention for your tuning in practice, such as cultivating intuition, deepening your connection with your inner guidance, or receiving clarity about a specific issue or question. Pay attention to any sensations, emotions, images, or thoughts that arise. Do not judge or analyze them; observe and allow them to flow through your awareness. Give yourself a minimum of ten or twenty minutes to listen. After you feel complete, take note of what you felt or received or any symbolic visions you may have had. Use your journal and see if anything else wants to come through around the topic.

Take some time to reflect on your experiences and interpret any symbols or messages you received. Consider how these insights may apply to your life or the intention you initially set. Keep in mind that the meanings may be allegorical, and your associations with the symbols or emotions can reveal insights.

Incilius alvarius

by Jana Cruder

10
Alchemical Mastery
When Integration Becomes Wisdom

*The one who is looking for knowledge is like an arrow shot
towards the Sun. If that arrow ever touches the Sun, it will
not come back; but if it touches the Sun and comes back to
Earth, it will no longer be an arrow.*

DOGON WISDOM

All altered states of consciousness help open us to other ways of looking at the world by getting us out of our normal cognition and into
a state of expanded awareness. Once in this place, we can see ourselves from a witness perspective, from our higher selves, and know
the truth of what we are. In these states, we can zoom out and connect to the separate parts of ourselves to integrate our psyche and our
soul into one whole self, a self that is more conducive to a joyful, free,
and peaceful existence.

The role of psychoactive plants and substances in this process is to remove the veil that separates us from the realm of Spirit,
to remind us that everything is connected, and to help bring up the
subconscious material to be composted within the psyche. The word
psychedelic—from the ancient Greek ψυχή (*psukhē*) and δῆλος (*dêlos*)—
means "manifest mind" or "evident spirit," according to Liddell and

Scott's *A Greek-English Lexicon*. As such, these medicines clear away perceptions of reality that the imprints of the egoic template have clouded, so we can see the truth: that the nature of life is mind-manifesting, relational, multidimensional, and interconnected.

The universal forces of nature and the cosmos desire for us all to have everything we want and need. We can all access doorways to the infinite life force within us, regardless of age, race, religion, or geography. If we can learn to trust this greater system at play and the ways to reach it, we can gradually open our potential to receive this gift. But modern society has forced other external systems that go against natural laws, traumatize us, and fill our heads with false beliefs, many of which impose limitations on our real power lying within. In the modern world, money has come to represent the power of life contained in both the forces of nature and within us. It has become the way we exchange manifestations of this life force. As such, many people now think of money as being synonymous with power. Within this system, life itself becomes a limited resource that is unevenly distributed among the population. But true power, life force energy, is not limited; only our conditioning and thinking tell us otherwise but it can be frightening to consider giving up these ways of being we've become so accustomed to. As doctor and poet Jaiya John warns, "Friends, do not enter this dance floor if you do not want to do this sacred dance. Everyone is losing their minds so they can remember their souls. And the only music playing is love."

A psychedelic experience is not a prerequisite to accessing this truth. Although, as we have seen, psychedelics are especially helpful in showing us our true natures because they amplify our patterns, allowing us to see more clearly how we behave in the world and whether this is working for or against us, and where the heart is open or closed. When individuals begin working with psychedelics for healing or growth, it is common for truth to be revealed rapidly, whether it comes from within oneself or from the outside world—*as within, so without.* Our dynamic interplay with these agents can accelerate the revelations telling us where we have blocks and where we need to do work internally.

Ultimately, the work of seeding consciousness is all in service of cultivating our creative power, the power within. Not what culture tells us power is, but real power, the kind that can never be taken from us because it is self-generating and comes from love. As our work here together comes to a close, this is what I really want you to understand—your inner abundance and your inner power, the agency created through compassion. All the chapters thus far have been leading up to this: how to recognize, cultivate, and use our power to create abundant lives that serve ourselves, our communities, and the Earth. The process of seeding consciousness centers around regular practice and refinement, making it integrative. Power is only cultivated through consistent, intentional practice. It starts with generous kindness toward yourself.

We also have great power as a collective. Still, we must first find our individual power and sovereignty so as to show up fully, without being driven by false motivations or relational patterns that perpetuate conflict or codependency. Further, we can't do other people's work for them. Everyone has their own work to do, and you can only do it for yourself. That doesn't mean we can't emotionally support our communities, families, and friends. It just means you must put on your oxygen mask before you help others. Do your work, find wholeness, and fully embody what you have learned. Doing your own work supports others, as others will witness your light, presence, and contentment and will be inspired to learn how you cultivated this resilience within yourself. As I said at the beginning of the book, heal yourself, and you'll heal the world without necessarily having to do anything. It is your way of being that will heal the world. Your light is the lantern for others in the times that we face. I believe this is true leadership.

Those who can recognize and understand the universal laws of nature—that the entire cosmos is reflected in both the three-dimensional plane and within ourselves—are innately the most prosperous because we can access the infinite power of the multiverse and create exactly the lives we want. I believe this makes us multidimensionaires! That is, each of us having some mastery or agency of our own energy and our hearts makes us, therefore, a force of nature in and of ourselves. Through this power, we can bring blessings to those close to us and do greater service for all of humanity.

The truth is that each of us has the ability to create our own reality. In fact we are doing so all the time, but many of us are creating from an unconscious place. Most of us may not realize that our thoughts, beliefs, and actions perpetually animate our reality in real time. We act from the unconscious mind; we don't see that we are attracting more of what is already inside us. As my mentor and early pioneer in psychedelic therapy Don Rosenthal said, "When I awaken from the dream, I can easily grasp the fact that I wrote the script and created the whole show. Every character was me in disguise. A bit more elusive in my waking dream, the same thing is true." When we understand the deeper truth of the universe and the forces of nature, we understand that the power to change our outward reality comes from within, not by forcing or doing, but with counsel and support from our guides, ancestors, nature, and the archetypal forces. As more of us learn these ancient teachings, we start to work at a higher expression, thereby expanding the collective consciousness's ability to co-create.

The purpose of seeding consciousness is cultivating our inner power, understanding how it works, and learning how to focus it in ways that directly benefit ourselves and others. In the previous chapters, I taught you about the various methods, practices, and cosmic side-roads that can help us on the journey. But now we are here, and this is where the true magic happens.

The Mastery Template

Having facilitated countless sessions with individuals in altered states of consciousness, I have observed an outpouring of creative expression following these inner explorations—poems, paintings, songs, books, and screenplays, all inspired by the experiences of people doing the inner work supported by non-ordinary states of consciousness. This tells me that when we reconnect to our souls in these realms through psychedelics and plant medicines, our creative energy flows more freely, untethered by the limitations of the egoic template.

When we are connected to our souls, we're naturally driven to create beauty in the world. I believe we are all creative beings, and the highest archetype we can embody is that of the Creative Master. This Master archetype personifies our highest potential, as exemplified by Kemet's neteru (gods). In no way do I want to put this idea on a pedestal that the ego can fluff itself up with. Renowned producer and creative Rick Rubin says, "You don't create greatness in search of an outcome, that's out of your control. Greatness comes from a practice of devotion." It is the archetype of the polymath, somebody who has developed a broad spectrum of worldly wisdom and mastery of practices, who is highly capable, an independent thinker, and conscientious of all life, dancing simultaneously between sovereignty and interbeing. Or the geisha, representing the ancient art of Japanese hospitality as an artist, healer, performer, conversationist, and host.

The notion that humans are here to embrace all knowledge and develop themselves as fully as possible is not a new idea. In ancient Kemet, one became part of society through initiation into a lifelong journey of refining one's own mastery of self. In the pharaonic times, the pharaohs had to go through lengthy preparations to become initiates before they were allowed to assume a leadership role. Imagine if this level of mastery of self was a prerequisite for anybody becoming a parent or running for office in modern-day government? Perhaps we would live in a society run by conscious adepts with more balance, compassion, and earth-connected leadership abilities.

The word *master* has some negative history because of its use in the context of slavery. This has caused many institutions to toss out the very word that represents the ultimate aim of alchemy. In light of this controversy, we must reclaim *master* for its sacred meaning. When I use this term, I mean it in the context of a guiding tenet or as a person who has refined their craft. On some level, though, everyone has a master, one that you have chosen consciously or unconsciously. Your master is either what you chase after—ego, power—or what you bow to in devotion to the great architect, the web of life. There is a cosmic order that must be followed and harmonized with to gain any level of mastery with oneself. Being a master is about being exalted or even being seen as such by others; it's about having agency over yourself. When you step into devotional service, you serve the greater whole and yourself. Masters humbly practice and refine themselves like works of art, through the most sacred act of purifying the heart.

In our own lives, we can embody the Master archetype when we access the collective unconscious and conscious wisdom through tuning in without being reactive and can wield and direct the untapped creative energy of the forces of nature. Rather than following the limiting dictates of the egoic template, we can live from our mastery template. This is when we engage with the final part of the inner alchemical process: the rubedo, where we take soul-embodied action out in the world. We've arrived at the final aspect of seeding consciousness—directing our creative power to embody numinous archetypal qualities in service to humanity, Earth, and all life.

When living from the mastery template, we are often called to some form of artistic expression, as art requires that we imitate nature; it is how we mirror what we learn from Earth, our collective mother. With each passing moment, Mother Earth creates works of art, and in each moment, she shares her creations with us. In many world religions such as Judaism, Christianity, and Islam, a primary attribute of the essence of God *is* Creator—or, we might say, the Grand Cosmic Artist or Architect. In these traditions, humans are created in God's image. Maybe what is implied is that we are a fractal of a larger intelligent cosmos, thus reflecting or mirroring the artistic capacities of this Grand Creative Force on a smaller scale.

Creativity doesn't have to be an artistic painting or music; any form of creative expression is meaningful. If you are in the business world, you can use your creativity to build a business that is an expression of your soul and nature's principles. If you are a nurse, your creativity can lead to innovative solutions and interventions that enhance your patients' well-being and support their recovery journey. This isn't just a conceptual idea; it's essential to life. It's not what you do but how you do it. Sometimes the most fun art is the kind that gets destroyed, like a nature altar, cooking, or sandcastle. Try playing with things that you know are going to be destroyed or decay, as it's one way of embracing creation in the face of change.

We must emulate nature, as the cycles of life and death or the natural order are where the real power exists. Anything we do that is not life-sustaining will not endure the test of time. It is destined to decay and fail. It is the natural law. Your career path or vocation doesn't matter as long as you are connected to something greater than simply making a living or making money and are acting from your wisdom of this natural order. If you're working for a paycheck, you are selling your true self short or just inviting upheaval and suffering to come your way. If you're working solely from the mind, there is only so much you can accomplish. It is through leading with your soul you connect to your creative power and feel truly fulfilled in life. This is an essential part of psychedelic integration and is the purpose of initiation.

When we are separated from the soul, this creative energy gets trapped and cannot be expressed clearly. It ends up manifesting instead as unhealthy desires, negative emotional build up, and the accumulation of power in the form of money and pursuit of material things. None of these drives are inherently wrong; when creativity is not fully expressed, the real issue is a self-imposed constriction of our inherent nature and the realization of our greatness and potential. Sometimes experiencing desire, addiction, or any of these expressions of pent-up creativity can be an integral part of the creative process and can teach us how to utilize our potential. The problem is that it leads to suffering and sickness in all forms when left unchecked, as the soul is suffocated. When fully activated and expressed, soul-based creation generates self-sustaining feelings of accomplishment and satisfaction, of being intrinsically connected and sharing our soul's gift with the greater whole.

Simply put, your soul is your connection to the universe and the information in the collective conscious. The mastery template, meanwhile, is the blueprint of your soul's greatest manifestation. It contains instructions for the highest expression of what your soul wants to create in this life. When we operate from the mastery template, we learn to recognize that the purpose of life is to love and create works of skill and beauty. So how do we begin to operate from the mastery template? One way is by using our intuition, or lunar self, to listen to our hearts. As we have seen, intuition communicates through emotion, using our feelings to guide us toward that which will illuminate and inspire us.

Ultimately, the difference between what you want for your life and what you manifest is whether you are empowering your egoic or mastery template. When approached with awareness, the mastery template shows us our capabilities in their highest ideal form, while the egoic template shows us the work we still have to do before we can manifest that reality. For instance, if you want to manifest a deeply connected relationship with a life partner, and you keep dating emotionally unavailable people, you may eventually realize that you have a core foundational belief lodged in the egoic template, a belief stating you're not worthy of a relationship in which both partners embrace openness and vulnerability. Because this is a place where you still have work to do, what you want in this area of your life will be different from what you manifest. The unconscious limiting belief rooted in the ego is the weed suffocating the beautiful seed of your conscious vision for your life.

When we are connected to the mastery template, we are not limited by inherited or ingrained ways of coping, or safety mechanisms that have become calcified and dysfunctional over time. As such, we can flow with life's tides by practicing deep acceptance of and surrendering to what is showing up rather than being reactive to it. And we can instead use that emotional energy to continually reorient ourselves toward living in a higher state, as a conduit of compassion. This is not always easy and tends to be a lifelong practice. Yet as we operate from this intentional way of being, we can continuously tap into the wisdom of both the universe and the innerverse, as mediated by the caring soul, to reveal what needs to be attended to in the present moment. Now, every decision we make and every action we take can bring us into greater alignment with the abundance and joy that is our true destiny.

Reaching our destiny requires us to take full responsibility for whatever happens in our lives, no matter what cards we've been dealt. As individuals, we have the power to transmute our shadows and move toward love. I am not saying this isn't hard or painful, or that you will excel at this straight out of the gate. Rather, we must accept and surrender as situations challenge us or push our growth edges. Such obstacles can feel like miniature forms of death and rebirth or ongoing cycles of destruction and transcendence. Whatever is showing up in your life is coming up for a reason—to teach you to be the Creative Master you came here to be, and to help your soul evolve. When we see things from that perspective, we can be less attached to specific outcomes and become witnesses to our experience. Even after reading this book, you may still struggle to accept that we live in a world of unspeakable suffering, trauma, and evil. Who would ever think that such horrific realities could fuel a positive or constructive process? Again, it goes back to the alchemical principles: the highest highs and the lowest lows exist because of their counterparts.

We must seek balance in all situations to get off this roller coaster. This balance can be found within ourselves. Just as a builder's level is used to create the perfect horizontal plane and balance, our connection with ourselves is a gauge that can help us ensure that our thoughts, deeds, and words are in check. As we become aware of the illusory nature of reality—as we experience it in some tangible way through mystical experiences—we become less reactive. Instead we learn to appreciate life, no matter what arises, and to have faith that all will be provided as we continue to confront the imprints of the egoic template and seed our consciousness with the wisdom of our souls. We can measure each moment against the next to orient with our highest soul alignment using the heart as our North Star.

The mastery template has qualities such as playfulness, curiosity, adventure, and self-empowerment that bring openness and receptivity to people, things, and situations. Nothing is labeled or assumed; all conflicts are welcomed. Conflict is recognized as an opportunity for reconciliation and healing. Above all, our greatest potential is always about feeling and expressing love and excitement—the art of creation—and sharing our unique gifts with the world.

Inner Alchemy and the Mastery Template

Now let's look at the role of seeding consciousness as the process of alchemy clears the path to access the mastery template. In any situation, you are either staying stuck in your egoic template by focusing on the fixed or looping patterns or behaviors (nigredo), or you are empowering your mastery template by tuning in to and listening to inner guidance (albedo). Only one of these can be given your power at any one time. Therefore we can only wield our creative life force energy through conscious action (rubedo) once we have engaged with the latter. And we can only do this once we have purged the blocks of the egoic template and become a vessel to tune in, receive, and listen to the soul.

As we have seen, alchemy is the art of transmutation: transforming one thing into another, into a purer and more transcendent form.

The alchemical process separates and reconstructs particular elements through a series of cleansing chemical processes. These reductions and restorations burn away impurities so that only a pure, refined essence remains. As such, the art of inner alchemy is a process of shedding light on the subconscious behaviors that have come to form the egoic template, and to make them conscious. This means getting to the root of the ego's desires, beliefs, and motivations, to discover where these are blocking access to our mastery template. Then we coagulate, which means bringing things back together or integrating them. This process of bridging the inner and outer worlds with the Spirit and the material realities is ongoing. It is the very meaning of my spiritual name, world-bridger.

As we have also learned, when applied to the self, inner alchemy requires us to progress through three phases that distill the ego into pure creative power (mastery):

Phase 1. Nigredo, representing where you are right now, or the thing you are trying to change.

Phase 2. Albedo, the act of tapping into your inner wisdom and pulling from your imagination and the spirit world to bring about change.

Phase 3. Rubedo, the actions needed to give rise to changes that align with your soul.

This process includes awareness of the ego (your reality) and the soul (your higher self), which will usher in the change you want to see in your life.

Nigredo

Phase one of engaging actively with the seeding consciousness process means clarifying your intentions. What do you want in life? What do you value? What do you want to create in the world, and why? The answers must come from your most authentic place. Question what you want and connect to the feeling of that thing, to ask if this is actually your highest possible aspiration and expression. For instance, if you want to manifest resources or prosperity for your life, endeavors, or community, you feel that in your body. You may realize that being abundant makes you feel powerful, so what you *really* want is power or to feel powerful. Or perhaps what you are seeking is support or provision from the universe. Maybe, instead of only seeking abundance, which may never actually satisfy you, you might think about other channels through which you can feel supported, empowered, or abundant.

Non-ordinary states of consciousness, whether induced by psychedelics, plant medicines, meditation, or journaling, can disrupt subconscious behaviors that hinder authentic desires. Surrendering to experiences outside our comfort zone may initially feel unnatural, but it's often the catalyst for profound inner transformation. For instance, exploring deep emotions like grief can unveil underlying subconscious patterns. Through this inner alchemical process, we confront and transmute these patterns, leading to greater freedom and self-realization.

In the context of alchemy, I like Irish playwright George Bernard Shaw's quote, "Life isn't about finding yourself. Life is about creating yourself." These experiences of confronting subconscious programming are essential in shaping the person you want to be. By delving into our inner landscape, we uncover hidden beliefs and traumas that shape our behaviors and perceptions. For example, recognizing the impact of early experiences, like a father figure's absence, can elucidate patterns of overexertion, self-sacrifice, and burnout. This nigredo, or state of darkness, must be acknowledged and transmuted to achieve greater authenticity and fulfillment.

Albedo

I have shown you here the literal process of converting the nigredo to the albedo—the fixed to the unfixed. The key is to focus on the specific area you have defined in Phase 1. Using the process of tuning in and connecting to the moon, ancestors, and your soul, you can start to tap into the albedo of the issue to receive information. Be sure to be open to as much information as possible, enough that it provides you with a feeling of understanding around the subject. Otherwise, it might need more time. If you feel stuck, go back to the nigredo step and make sure you are honing your understanding of what this situation actually is. Also, hold the situation lightly—be wary of paralysis by analysis.

Ultimately, the best approach may involve a combination of modalities. Choosing a path often depends on your time and resources, as well as the depth of the blockage. You might meditate to gain initial insights, explore deeper issues through plant medicine ceremonies, bringing in forgiveness, and journal about your experiences to integrate the lessons and revelations. The key is to remain open to multiple methods and adapt your approach based on your needs, preferences, and circumstances. Sometimes just sitting with something intentionally, giving the situation part of yourself, your emotion or your presence, can create a decisive shift in energy. Take it slowly. There is no need to rush, ever.

Rubedo

Only once we understand what we want authentically, from our limitless soul, and what is blocking us, from our finite ego, are we free to choose to empower ourselves. Remember, you empower one or the other with every choice you make. You choose to love (soul) or fear (ego) every moment. Continuing to empower your mastery template (rubedo) is an ongoing practice of not allowing the mind to project egoic conditioning onto your experiences, and engaging with life exactly as it is, without judgment.

We all have free will. In each moment, we choose which part of ourselves runs the show: will it be the ego or our mastery over it? While this notion may seem simple, we often need daily help with this face-off. Many times, the voices of our inner critic and other inner guardians are so loud and ingrained that we continue to follow their nudges without question. From my experience in witnessing journey-work over and over, the biggest internal issue that we have as a species is the fear of our own power. Why would we fear our power? We may fear our power because of early trauma-based conditioning or expectations set by society or our families, which have kept us stuck or paralyzed in frozen states of unworthiness, inadequacy, self-doubt, fear of failure, perfectionism, or overwhelm, leaving us questioning our true capacity and infinite potential. This fear causes us, the egoic template, to clamp down and try to control things, blocking access to our mastery template. To illuminate what is holding you back, all you must do is listen to the negative dialogues or emotions. Try writing them down as you experience them and track them for patterns.

Aligning with the mastery template through inner alchemy means seeing every challenge as a creative opportunity. The mastery template doesn't contain self-imposed barriers or limitations of the ego. The creative master within sees a wall and says, "No worries! I'll just take a helicopter." As philosopher Jean Gebser poetically said, "Don't forget this, these walls have yet another side: these things which seem immovable to you are full of transformation."

The fruits of the seeding consciousness process grow in bountiful ways, as we align with our mastery template. This is when we start to move through the process naturally, and it becomes part of how we approach the world. Remember, alchemy is about turning base metal into gold. Gold is the metal corresponding to the Sun. The Sun is the ultimate carrier of prana, the energy that permeates every living thing. When we are in our mastery template, we re-source from the lunar depths of the soul to become our own abundant, self-sustaining source of this energy. We become sovereign over our inner domain and can direct our creative energy most potently. The ego becomes a vehicle for our creative expression rather than the source of our suffering. Our touch becomes like Midas, turning things around us into gold.

When we live in harmony with our creative potential, we expend very little energy and instead *receive* energy continuously from the great web of life, allowing for a simple and free manifestation process. In Eastern philosophy, they call this *wu wei*, the place of effortless action. As such, operating through the mastery template enables us to tap into an endless energy source and open ourselves up to our limitless potential.

Mastering Our Power

Remember how, when I described the process of inner alchemy at the beginning of the book, I shared an example of how I used this process to work on my money blocks? I chose this story intentionally. As stated above, in the modern world, money has become synonymous with power—and to tap into our creative wellspring, we first need to understand the true meaning of power, what it is, and where it comes from. This also means understanding what it is *not*: that is, money, fame, or being the CEO of a successful company. True power is self-awareness. It is being in flow and knowing that the universe is abundant and ready to offer everything you need with each intentional step. It knows that you have the power to co-create your own reality. As I have stated, this is our birthright, no matter who you are, where you come from, or what has happened in your past.

So how is it that power came to be represented by money and has been distributed so unevenly in the world? In ancient cultures, such as the Nuer of Sudan, a man's wealth was measured by his cattle and women (for the Nuer, specifically through dowry, a marriage agreement made through exchange of cattle), because cows and women generate *life*. Life and wealth were one and the same. The Kemetic cow-headed goddess Hathor, who represents the principle of fertility and is ruled by the planet Venus and the metal copper, was one of the most revered gods. Hathor symbolizes the archetype of the mother, love, beauty, and music. Venus represents the feminine, or the creative force, associated with material abundance. Copper is also a superconductor of energy, meaning energy moves freely. Simply put, before the invention of money, "wealth" was synonymous with creativity and generativity—or how we each manifested the life force flowing through us in the world.

Now I'm not saying we should return to a system where cows and women represent value. To return to a belief in our own power to generate inner and outer abundance, we must return to the idea that real wealth lies in becoming superconductors of creative energy and creating value by supporting life.

The ancients also knew that the Earth was the source of all wealth, whether it be food, water, or the air we breathe. They knew their relationship with the great Mother determined how prosperous they would be, and so they gave offerings to the land, cared for the soil, and performed rituals to bring abundant rain. When we embody the feminine and act as stewards and caregivers of the land, the soil, and the ocean, it creates more abundance for all life on this planet. In contrast, our extractive capitalist culture and the financial systems that drive it are based on myopic, short-term goals that pollute our air, water, and soil and put the value of people, animals, and nature secondary to money and go against the concept of us each being part of a vast, interconnected web of life.

In our modern era, we need to remember that all life flows from Earth. Rather than accept the air, water, and food as nature's gift to us, we began to extract the oil and gold from her veins. Then, human beings put price tags on things that were given freely to them. Over many centuries of this practice, the Western monetary system came to be based on the false premise that *life itself* can be bought, whether in the form of the Earth's natural resources or the hours of our lives that we exchange for a paycheck. But the money that existed long before the fiat currencies we use now was asset-backed notes and gold. The first banks formed when families made pilgrimages and needed a place to keep their possessions safe. Although banking can be traced to ancient Mesopotamia, banks began to serve a central role in American society during the mid 1800s, when banks like Wells Fargo formed to hold the gold mined during the California Gold Rush. Rather than carrying gold, people used notes or certificates, which were far more portable and could be exchanged for gold at any time. Only in 1933 did President Roosevelt do away with the "gold standard" in the United States, which led to the use of the fiat currency we use today.

As we have seen, gold is symbolic of more than just currency. For the people of Kemet and the alchemists of old, gold was representative of our highest creative potential and was associated with metamorphosis and personal transformation. It was the result of the alchemical process of transmuting dense matter to something finer. To the alchemists, gold represents our personal power and innate self-sovereignty, as held in our solar plexus chakra. Therefore owning gold or being "wealthy" represents maintaining personal sovereignty, both on a physical and metaphysical level.

As such, banks and governments took away our sovereignty using fiat currencies. Now many government entities, such as the Federal Reserve in the United States, can essentially print as much money as they want. This can majorly impact inflation, devaluing every dollar of currency that people hold in savings or other assets. Banks can make money appear from nowhere, through derivatives of saving deposits, which loans they issue, and charging interest. This gives the banks massive power to leverage their customers' money—in other words, it gives them sovereignty. And who ends up owning the asset the bank loaned against if you can't pay? The bank!

We live in a system that creates promissory notes that no longer hold true to their promise of being redeemable in gold bullion. But this currency must have some life force behind it, or the system would not function. Do you know what that life force is? It's you. Since our power comes from where we put our attention and resources, when its focus is outside of us, it can empower systems that grow at a massive scale and that greatly harm the planet and its people.

Over time, banks have imposed rules and passed laws through collusion with governments, eroding individuals' sovereignty over their finances and thus their creative power. In many ways, this *is* the separation wound that so many of those who come to me for healing are suffering from. Why are we putting our precious seeds in other people's storehouses and allowing them to control how we can plant them? The tragedy is that we have become dependent on these systems that have no mercy or compassion for any living being. The only way to reclaim sovereignty over our creative power is to seed our consciousness with insights, wisdom, and beliefs that remind us of our true, innate abundance and create new systems. Let's diversify and plant seeds in places where we want to grow, and let's have reciprocal relationships that nurture and sustain us. That might be in land, farms, communal ownership of goods. . . . Suppose we continue to empower corporate greed—which in many ways represents the collective egoic template—rather than elevating ourselves to become leaders who embody the principles of natural law. How will we ever disrupt the status quo?

Money is a social construct based on our agreed-upon societal values. But we have gone from a system reliant on the ownership of cows, and then gold, to a system essentially backed by nothing other than what we believe or give value to. Unlike cows (or women), today's money has no value in and of itself; we are the ones who give it value through our creative efforts. In a system that rewards creativity, the power will always reside with those who have their fingers on the pulse of the real needs of society. Therefore the way to reclaim our power is to begin to live again from the mastery template. When our creative contributions match the true needs of the collective, as opposed to the fear-based wants of a society bred on scarcity, we discover that the great web of life will naturally provide for everything we need.

Alchemizing Gold

Returning to placing our trust in life is easier said than done. The monetary system described above is difficult to detach from because we carry much collective trauma around safety and belonging as a species—a result of having been severed from our sovereignty and creative power. This fear is easily activated by media messaging around scarcity, polarization, and alienation. And when humans are driven by fear, we react by rushing off and stockpiling toilet paper. Competition and greed have become the norm.

Instead, when we want to better understand our relationships to money, power, and creativity or to manifest more of each, we might ask the question, "To what purpose might I dedicate myself to become a conduit for resources to flow through, for myself and others, and for the highest good of the planet?" This framing infuses our relationship to money with the power of our own souls. We can also look at the alchemical principles to understand our inner power and creative energy, which is our true gift to the world and is what we came here to offer. But before you can use your power and gifts in service, you must clear out the muck blocking you from realizing that power. Practices for doing so are described throughout this book.

Let me show you a final example of this work in practice. I remember meeting a magical woman who inspired me to shift my perspective on my own creative potential—and therefore my financial abundance. She was an artist and die-hard Burner—a regular attendee of the annual Burning Man festival—who, I noticed, was incredibly generous to her friends. Her generosity inspired me, and I gently inquired about her story. She shared that she'd been having a hard time making money and didn't understand why. During an ayahuasca ceremony, she asked, "How can I manifest massive wealth and prosperity?" This question addressed her limitations when it came to manifesting, and her clear desire to be aligned in service and with nature in the way she provided for herself and in how she shared her gifts and her heart with the world. The message from the medicine was that if she was to manifest this money, she had to balance her energy about money to keep the power from having negative karma attached to it.

She was also told that she must bless any money that came her way, so that it would create good in the world. After the initiation, she meditated on this answer, turning to her lunar side for insights (albedo). Then she came up with a plan (rubedo): every time she bought something for herself, she would give someone the same amount. So that's what she did. When she got a massage, she also gifted an unsuspecting friend a massage. When she went out to dinner, she treated someone. Every time, she used her intuition to feel what and to whom she was to give.

Rather than being a magic trick to get more money for herself, this all came from a deeply authentic place and represented a letting go of the scarcity mindset that had kept her stuck. And as she got the hang of this process, the money started to pour in for her. Sometimes she was making $40,000 in a month with her business. And each time she brought in physical cash, she did a ceremony on the money, smudging it and using a blacklight stamp to bless each bill before sending it back into the world on its future journey. Finally, she prayed and thanked the universe and the spirits for the blessings of this wealth and abundance in her life. After she invested in a beautiful home, she gifted one of the bedrooms to an artist friend to help them get on their feet. She did this for several years until she bought a farm and worked the land, retiring from her abundance practice. Now she shares her gifts with the world, doesn't worry about how to pay her bills or sustain herself, collects eggs from her chickens, and picks fresh vegetables from her garden.

Returning to the alchemical process, her nigredo was the limitations in her mindset about creating resources or money for herself so that she could be fully aligned with her soul's desire to be in service.

The albedo was to ask the medicine, her intuition, and the spirit realm for support on how to transmute this old unconscious belief structure, and then crafting the plan she created based upon the information she received from the medicine. The rubedo was putting it into action, step by step.

She also balanced her Sun and Moon, action and stillness, and effort and inner guidance throughout the process. But most importantly, she began to view money as the alchemists might: as energy and potential. She then connected to her creative power and sovereignty by doing something counterintuitive—inviting in flow by giving it away—to increase her capacity for abundance. Most importantly, she rebuilt trust in her creative power, not just for herself but for the benefit and service of others. Although she didn't explicitly state it, she understood again that we do not earn money or abundance; we create it.

Remember, alchemy is about turning base metal into gold. Gold is the metal corresponding to the Sun, the ultimate carrier of the prana that animates every living thing. When we are in our mastery template, we become the source of that energy in a metaphysical sense. Living in that mastery template makes us naturally empowered and abundant. In a way, we *are* the money. We are wealth itself because our internal power manifests externally as self-sustaining abundance. It is our consciousness that allows it to manifest. We have regained our power by making the internal shifts needed to erode the old beliefs or blocks.

But it doesn't end there. In order to express your inner Creative Master, you have to keep on creating gold from your highest truth. This process has become second nature for me. Now whenever I take on a new creative project, I tune in and clarify what I want to birth through me, and I constantly refine the process to get as clear as possible on my intention. When a block comes up, I meditate on it and get more information about the block. I go within, ask many questions, and wait until the answers arise. I use the divination tools in the chapter about tuning in to see if I get the same information over and over from a multitude of converging sources or if new information arises. Through this process, I can see where my work is aligned with my path and my place in the greater order. I am constantly readjusting my strategy based on information from my intuition and what shows up, to ensure I am working for my highest good and the highest good of all.

The more you play an active role in your creative manifestation, digging deeper into what's going on at all levels, the more metaphysical gold you will create in your life. As you align each part of yourself through the alchemical process, you weave the fabric of creation, which is your life. But I hope you understand that this conversation isn't about money at all; it's about creating spiritual and personal power, most importantly through receiving instructions that lie outside of purely self-centered motivation. It is in devotion to service and all life. What's not good for life is not good for you. Inner alchemy is the process of empowering ourselves to move energy more consciously. Mastery is about following the golden thread, kundalini or life force energy that animates all things, moving through the web of life to create change through the forces of nature. We can practice our instinctual ability to move away from what life no longer supports and toward what is coming into manifestation, by attuning our senses to where the creative energy is going and how to follow it. This is where we can, with practice, easily let go of attachments and grievances, and find comfort in the liminality of not knowing. We can work with the laws of nature to transform the leaden parts of our lives into gold by redistributing the energy from the ego and feeding it back to empower the soul through discipline-focused attention or agency. Thus we plant the seeds for abundance and freedom in our lives and the lives of others.

The flourishing psychedelic renaissance shows how many of us are ready and willing to engage with this work. A shift in focus has taken place, with society as a whole orienting toward seeding consciousness.

My highest hope for this movement is that it finds more and more of us stepping out of scarcity and engaging with our full creative potential from an empowered place fueled by our souls. Then we will divest from the extractive practices that have wrought such havoc on our Earth, our home. We must step into the mystery. We must learn to trust phenomena that can't always be explained by science, like the spirit world and intuition. We must be willing to go into the darkness, let our egos die, and to lean deep into our shadows. We will then reclaim our rightful role as stewards, guardians of nature, and masters of the cosmic forces that are the architecture all of life.

Liberation

As we delve deeper into our inner work, how can we discern whether we've traversed it successfully or attained any degree of mastery? I find there are intriguing parallels between Bwiti and the concept of liberation that offer some clues. Within Bwiti, there's a rich symbolism centered on the harmonization of dualities, such as the balance between masculinity and femininity represented by the colors white and red (see page 122). It's striking to note that the capital city of Gabon, the birthplace of Iboga, bears the name Libreville, meaning "free town."

The initiation rites of women in the Fang tradition of Bwiti give more evidence for this connection. Adorned in white togas and holding torches fashioned from okoume tree resin, adorned with plant crowns, they evoke the iconic imagery of the Statue of Liberty. It's intriguing to consider the significance of France—the nation that bestowed the Statue of Liberty upon the United States—being home to artists like Picasso, Henri Matisse, and André Breton who were collectors of Bwiti artifacts. It was rumored that prominent artists and luminaries clandestinely engaged with iboga, and even the prestigious fashion label Hermès produced a scarf featuring traditional Bwiti masks, suggesting subtle influences interwoven into the very threads of French culture.

Liberty has been a controversial topic since the day it arrived in New York. Frédéric Auguste Bartholdi, the artist chosen to create the Statue of Liberty, had experiences in Egypt that may have influenced the monument's design, potentially incorporating elements that point to mystical underpinnings.

It wouldn't be too far off to consider the Statue of Liberty holds some symbolism in the potency of initiation.

Within the journey toward liberation, there are discernible markers that signify that phases of initiation have occurred:

Stage 1. Uninitiated

In this stage, life appears to happen to you. You experience existence through a lens of resistance, conflict, and often victimhood. Your reactions and perceptions are heavily influenced by personal, societal, and inherited traumas. At times, the world seems chaotic and beyond your control, leading to feelings of powerlessness, anger, or frustration.

Stage 2. Initiate

As you progress, you begin to see life as happening for you rather than to you. Here, you begin to perceive life's experiences as reflective mirrors, integrating the lessons learned. The individual agency led by the soul allows you to choose rather than feeling the need to be in control or have domain over others. Personal agency becomes a driving force, allowing you to navigate and influence your surroundings with increasing skill. You start to view life as a learning process, with Earth as your classroom for soul evolution. Instead of seeking control, you learn to make conscious choices aligned with your inner wisdom.

Stage 3. Master

In this advanced stage, you realize that life happens through you. You surrender fully to the flow of existence, becoming a conduit for consciousness itself. Your actions stem from a soul-led orientation rather than ego-driven reactions or desires. You embody a state of allowing, where you harmoniously respond with the greater currents of life. Your presence becomes a catalyst for transformation, effortlessly influencing your environment and others around you. This phase is marked by complete surrender. You become a vessel through which consciousness flows.

Throughout these stages, you evolve from a reactive participant to an active co-creator. Each phase builds upon the last, representing a deepening understanding of your role in the cosmic dance of existence. This is a rough map, as there is commonly a blending of one stage to another as parts of oneself integrate through practice.

In Bwiti tradition, individual liberation is found through initiation, where individuals confront themselves and delve into the roots of their suffering. Through this process, they emancipate themselves to acknowledge the inherent power within. Subsequently they integrate into the broader community, extending support to others on their paths to liberation through similar processes. The hermetic principle "as above, so below" underscores that by liberating ourselves, we widen the gateway for collective liberation. When one is initiated in Gabon, they are paraded around town by their nima and everyone celebrates the new member of the community. You are not born into Bwiti, and it is seen as moving up in society when you complete your first stage of initiation to become a Bwitist.

Mycelial Perspective

I leave you with this final thought: whether we're healing ourselves or the planet, we cannot do it alone. We need each other. The mycelium, the vegetative part of a fungus, is a great teacher of how teamwork and the dissolution of self may expand the capacity for all life to thrive. The mycelium starts off as spores; the spores spread amongst the forest and grow hypha, little tiny roots that all grow together to form a vast mycorrhizal network that permeates the entire forest. Mycelia are the distributors of resources. They help the forest to communicate in order to remove decaying matter or facilitate the transport of nitrogen, carbon, and other minerals to parts of the forest that need support. Literally, the mycelium is brokering the exchanges between trees that are healthy and ones that are in need of additional sugars for photosynthesis—they are the helpers of the forest and maintain the balance of nature. Energy must flow freely for life to thrive, and the mycelium feeds on decomposing matter to create new growth. Mushrooms are the ultimate alchemists. That is why taking psilocybin mushrooms reminds us of our interdependence with all life. We can glean wisdom from our fungal friends and take down borders to become a network that elevates the well-being of all forms of life.

The mycelium provides a valuable lesson about teamwork and the dissolution of self, demonstrating that by working together and prioritizing the needs of the community, all life can thrive. When we let go of our self-centered worries and instead focus on serving others and the greater whole, we discover that our own needs are naturally met, and we experience greater happiness and connection with ourselves and those around us. The mycelium teaches us the importance of maintaining balance and stepping into service for the benefit of all.

A healthy community is just like a mycelial network in the forest, helping to spread resources and nutrients to the places that are most in need. It is no wonder that when one takes psilocybin mushrooms, the mushrooms act like a mycelial network inside your brain, imbuing an intelligence to the neurons within oneself that point to precisely where the broken connections are, thus reminding us of the interdependence of all of life. These little teachers show us that we need to be in balance with ourselves, others, and our environment, or we suffer the consequences of disconnection and dis-ease.

By exploring our inner selves, we can gain some degree of orientation in this realm of the unknown. However, this process primarily involves letting go of control and surrendering to the mystery. It can be disorienting, and sometimes the message is unclear, as if transmitted through a television with a poorly tuned antenna. We delve into our inner selves to understand who we are, so we can live authentically on this Earth. These mystical experiences can help us to relax and not take our material reality too seriously, or at least realize there's a lot more happening under the soil.

As the altered state subsides and we descend down the mountain of the peak experience, we may feel that we're back where we started, which can lead to a sense of despair. Psychedelic integration is about taking the awareness we open during these non-ordinary states and grounding it into our physical world, allowing us to embody a more deliberate consciousness and way of being. While we may gain intelligence through a mystical experience, being able to use it as a resource in your daily life is a different matter. Sometimes one who has experienced these mystical states thinks they carry the wisdom of it—but they have yet to integrate the knowledge from it. There's still work to do, and what they've uncovered needs to be properly digested. This is the phase or cycle during which you need to allow time for the world to reflect back the new framework seeding within you. How do you know you've actually changed unless you respond differently to life? This reflection back from community and the world is an essential mirror to orient you on your journey.

Sure, the road may not be an easy one, but now that you are initiated into seeding consciousness, why keep on the path? As Ram Dass said in his book *Be Here Now*: "Once the Seed has been planted—once you have been born again—you don't have a choice." These wonderous and complex systems in nature and the cosmos have so much yet to teach and offer you. Psychedelics and plant medicines are ready and willing to support us in the work we need to do to move forward. Know that the psychedelics and plant medicines alone will not rescue us from the work each and every one of us must do, but they are great allies for fostering resilience, connection, and our own creative empowerment.

We've covered a lot of ground. As I said in the beginning, not all of what's presented here will land for you. It could take time, and certain lessons may never work for your situation. That's okay. Do you have unanswered questions? That might mean there is some homework to do.

· · · · · · · · · · · · · · ·

SEEDING CONSCIOUSNESS IN PRACTICE

Intention Connection

Let's start by tapping back into the skills of tuning in; let's connect to your soul, the ancestors, or archetypal symbols such as the Sun or Moon. The exercise may help you explore and address any unanswered questions or sources of uneasiness related to the material covered, by tuning in to your soul, connecting with your ancestors, or engaging with the archetypal energies of the Sun or Moon.

Find a quiet and comfortable space where you won't be disturbed. Sit or lie down in a relaxed position and take a few deep breaths to center yourself. Close your eyes and continue to connect to your breath.

As you breathe and focus on your inner intelligence, set an intention to connect with it, or with your ancestors, or an archetypal energy such as that of the Sun or Moon. You can do this by silently making a request or simply holding the intention in your heart. Once you feel connected, bring to mind any unanswered questions or points of unease related to seeding consciousness. What points cause you uneasiness? What part of seeding consciousness is not taking root for you? Hold these questions in your awareness and allow yourself to be open to any insights, messages, or guidance that may come through.

Be patient and give yourself time to listen to and observe any sensations, emotions, or thoughts that arise. Stay present and receptive, allowing the connection to unfold naturally. When you feel ready to end the practice, take a moment to express gratitude to your soul, ancestors, or the archetypal energy you connected with. Slowly open your eyes and return to your surroundings.

Take some time to reflect on the insights or messages you received during the practice. You may wish to journal about your experience to help integrate any newfound clarity or understanding.

Remember, this practice can be repeated as often as needed to explore any lingering questions or areas of discomfort. By continually tuning in and connecting to these sources of wisdom and guidance, you can deepen your understanding of the material and foster a greater sense of connection with the wisdom that lies within and around you.

Sometimes with psychedelics and plant medicines, these unsettling places are an opportunity to find stillness. To be capable of holding complexity comes from being complete and whole, yet at the same time embracing what is uncertain, unknown, or incomplete—just as the Moon is always whole but you may only see one phase of it. This is part of the path. This liminal space is a place for patience and compassion. One of the greatest gifts we can give ourselves is to spend even a second here and find some sense of grounding. This is a lifelong journey of many cycles of deaths and rebirths. As my late mentor, Malidoma Patrice Somé, said, "See the journey and the destination as one and the same." That is what creativity truly is!

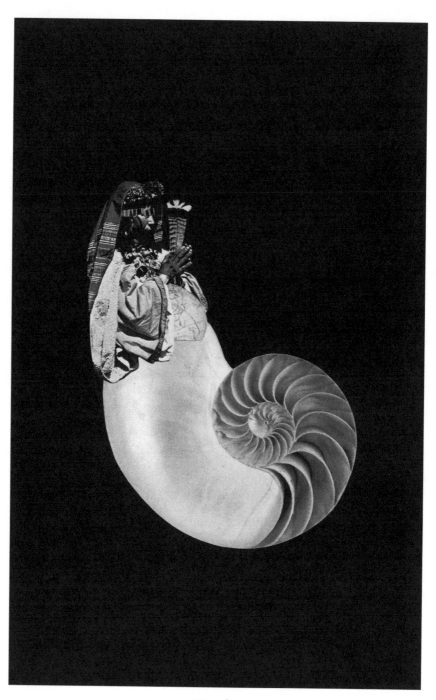

Nautilus

by Ashley Edes

APPENDIX 1

The Wisdom Keepers

I am honored to present the mentors and teachers to whom I've looked for guidance, who have also recorded a great body of wisdom in books and documentaries that you can find and learn from yourself. Although this book I've written came from instructions I received in one of my initiations in Gabon, and is written from my soul, my elders guided me as I frequently checked in to ensure I was sharing things properly and accurately. In the spirit of transparency and integrity, it is important to note here that this doesn't mean I am representing any tradition, speaking for any lineage, or suggesting that any of these elders endorse every word I say, unless they specifically provided their endorsement within these pages. Their influence is ever-present, but the book itself is about a process that bridges the Western world and original principles, a process I discovered within myself. This book is a representation of my understanding of the original principles in practice, from my personal experience, which is supported by anthropological evidence and anecdotal accounts. I always am respectful of any elders' time, knowing the demands of their life missions and old age that cause limitations in their lives. I have provided financial compensation for any requests for help with this book, even though these wisdom keepers always give generously of their time and expect nothing in return. The author proceeds from the book will go to support each one of these wisdom keepers' great missions on Earth and above. My NGO, Ancestral Heart, will continue to support all of these wisdom keepers in addition to numerous other projects. As well, many of these elders have entire villages and teams supporting them. The villagers and team members all play some role in the healing and teaching, so I honor them, too, as I acknowledge each wisdom keeper. I also acknowledge the organizations for which I have sat in council and that have gathered many of these elders: Holistic Visions, Le Ceil Foundation, Alliance for the Sacred Sites of Earth Gaia (ASSEGAIA), Earthrise Collective, The Fountain, and my nonprofit, Ancestral Heart.

My prayer is that this book will inspire you to also support our collective mission in some way, either through Ancestral Heart or by giving directly to the organizations listed on each elder's dedicated page. It doesn't matter how much one gives; it's the expression of reciprocity that matters. Of course, if you have the means and feel inspired, it would be the greatest honor to see these wisdom keepers be lifted up.

Due to current regulations on psychedelics in certain countries, some of my elders who regularly travel wished not to be mentioned here for the sake of security, as some countries, such as France, have harsh penalties for even suspected activities related to the sacraments that some of these elders work with. I intend to support them on a more discreet, individual level out of respect for their wishes for privacy.

Rutendo Lerato Ngara

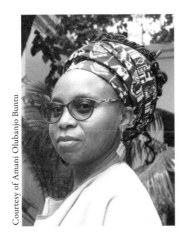

Courtesy of Amani Olubanjo Buntu

Region: South Africa

Wisdom Tradition: Zulu

Organizations: Credo Mutwa Foundation, Ancestral Heart

Rutendo Ngara is an African Indigenous Knowledge Systems practitioner and transdisciplinary researcher whose professional interests have spanned from clinical engineering, healthcare technology management, socio-economic development, mathematics, leadership, and fashion design to the interface between science, culture, cosmology, nature, and paradigms of healing.

Ngara is a co-founder of Ancient Wisdom Africa and the Ancient Wisdom Foundation, and coordinator of the Earthrise Collective, an international coalition weaving together ancient wisdom with activism and building alternative world systems. She serves on a number of boards and advisory committees, including the Credo Mutwa Foundation (chairperson), the ASSEGAIA Alliance, the Indigenous Knowledge Systems for Heritage Animals Council, the South African Wushu Federation, the People's World Commission on Drought and Flood (commissioner), and Ancestral Heart.

Ngara consults in transdisciplinary research and has worked in website management, research and development in the clinical engineering and healthcare technology management arenas, and has taught mathematics, English, African spirituality, and science. She has served in research and research coordinator roles at the University of Cape Town and UNISA.

She holds a B.S. in electrical engineering and an M.S. in medicine in biomedical engineering, and also holds a number of certificates including English language teaching and a fashion design diploma. She is pursuing a transdisciplinary doctorate.

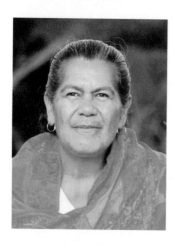

Atarangi Murupaenga

Region: Aotearoa/New Zealand
Wisdom Tradition: Ahipara
Organization: Māori Healers

Atarangi is a revered knowledge and lineage holder, inheriting her wisdom from the teachings of her various Aunts, including Pearl Allen, Bella Nathan, Heniwera Phillips, and Whaea Skipper. In the literal translation of her name, *ata* means "dawn" and *rangi* means "light," representing a vibration or energy. In the old language, *atarangi* signifies "the realization of one's visions," in the words of Naida Glavish.

Her tribal affiliations encompass Ngati Kuri and Te Aupouri from her father's side and Te Rarawa and Ngati Pakahi from her mother's side. The wealth of knowledge she possesses has been enriched by figures like Papa Joe, Manu Korewha, Makuini Ruth Tai, and Rose Pere, as well as her grandparents and *whanau* (family).

Atarangi's approach to healing is elegantly simple, utilizing *raakau* (types of sticks), *kohatu* (stones), and leaves from certain trees. Despite its simplicity, the work carries profound depth due to her understanding of how to employ these tools effectively.

Teachings like Mahi Raakaau, focused on self-help and self-healing, were common in the households of the tribal villages in the Northern New Zealand. The human body was likened to a *whare* or house, and when someone expressed feelings of *mamae* (pain), the healer had an innate understanding of how to address it.

Atarangi's passion for the healing arts was ignited by her elders, who initiated her training at a young age. Like many of her time, she learned from the esteemed *kaumātua* (elders), and the potency of their teachings is evident in her healing work.

Atarangi, or Ata, as she is known, has been sharing her teachings across the globe for more than two decades. Her dedication lies in the healing arts that belong to the realm and teachings of the Divine Feminine. This entails sharing specific knowledge with different age groups; for instance, she imparts wisdom to young girls aged eight to twelve (*kotiro taitamariki*), teaching them how to nurture their bodies with exercises to prepare them for their first cycles. This way, they embrace this significant phase with a sense of calm and understanding, honoring their rights and rite of passage. Atarangi extends these healing arts to her children, grandchildren, and extended family, both biological and spiritual.

Jyoti Ma

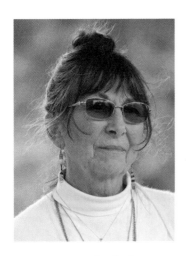

Region: California, United States
Wisdom Tradition: Multiple
Organization: The Fountain
Website: The Fountain Earth

Jyoti Ma (Jeneane Prevatt), Ph.D., is an internationally renowned spiritual teacher. As the spiritual director of the Center for Sacred Studies, she co-founded Kayumari, which has spiritual communities both in America and Europe. Other projects she has helped to convene are the International Council of Thirteen Indigenous Grandmothers and the Unity Concert. She is the founder of The Fountain, whose mission is to restore an economic model that is based on reciprocity and collaboration guided by Nature and the Sacred.

Jyoti has devoted her life to bringing unity to the planet by facilitating the development of alliances between individuals who are the guardians of Indigenous culture and traditional medicine ways. Through this work, collaborative relationships with organizations focused on economic, social, and environmental solutions have developed, creatively addressing the global challenges of our times. Jyoti has a B.A. in education from Northwestern State University in Natchitoches, LA; an M.A. in Human Relations and Community Affairs from the American International College in Springfield, MA; and a Ph.D. in transpersonal psychology with a special emphasis on cross-cultural aspects of spiritual development in children and adults from Summit University in New Orleans. She took postgraduate studies at the C. G. Jung Institute in Switzerland.

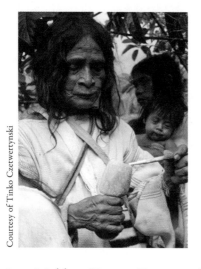

Courtesy of Tinko Czetwertynski

Kogi Mamo Luis Nuevita Jandingua

Region: Sierra Nevada de Santa Marta, Colombia
Wisdom Tradition: Kogi Kággaba
Organizations: Nativa Foundation, Ancestral Heart

Mamo Luis is a revered Kogi Kággaba mamo, a spiritual leader among the Kogi people. Mamo Luis was born into Mukhua Kungui Ezuama village.

At the age of five he began the formation in darkness in the Ezuama of Sezhangajrha, one of the Kogi's most sacred sites. Each mamo has a unique role, and Mamo Luis is known as the Son of the Sun. Some of his areas of knowledge are the mystical governance of gold, the ancient Kággaba language, and mask work with sacred objects passed down to Kogi Ancestors. When Mamo Luis became an adult, he received *poporo* in the Kabusankhua sacred site. The poporo is a sacred object imbued with cultural and spiritual meaning for the Kogi Kaggaba mamos. It is a gourd that is consecrated by ceremony for the mamos to carry. They mix the coca leaf or "ayu" (which means mother) and lime which they chew on. The poporo represents the womb of mother and the way of mixing and praying with the ayu opens the channels mamos to fulfill their commitment to be in balance with her (nature).

Mamo Luis became, essentially, an ambassador, traveling worldwide to remind humanity of its responsibility as stewards of the Earth. He works to reactivate the planet's natural sacred sites, which help maintain balance across all ecosystems. Considered one of the longest-lived mamos who is still alive and active, he has for more than 100 years been part of the institutional creation of the Gonawindúa Tayrona Organization, together with the great enlightened leaders Jacinto Zaragata and Pedro Juan Nuevita, now deceased. The Gonawindúa Tayrona Organization is the representative body of the Kággaba government and the legitimate institution that represents the Kággaba people before the Colombian state and society.

Mamo Luis has appeared in the documentary *Aluna*, which highlights the Kogi Kággaba people, as well as the 2019 film *The Twelve: A Tale of Wisdom and Unity*. The latter film follows twelve elders chosen to form a wisdom council and perform a unifying prayer for humanity to live in love and harmony with one another and the natural world.

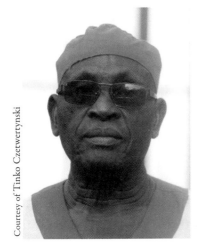

Courtesy of Tinko Czetwertynski

Atome Ribenga

Region: Gabon
Wisdom Tradition: Bwiti Fang
Organization: Le Ciel Foundation

Maitre Atome Ribenga has served as a consecrated priest in the Bwiti tradition for fifty years. Bwiti is one of the oldest ancestral traditions using iboga as part of its initiatory rites.

Through Master Atome's studies of monotheism and theology, he discovered his life's mission—helping people to reconnect with the Spirit and the divine within themselves. In full humility, with inexhaustible curiosity for the cosmos, he teaches so as to give people an opportunity to learn on their own, through direct experience, so they can discover their inner truth and not a written one. Master Atome spent his life tirelessly contributing to his spiritual tradition, including writing nine books on Bwiti, in French.

Atome's efforts, arising from his deep dedication to his spiritual work, are the inspiration behind the film *The Twelve*, which shares the wisdom of twelve spiritual elders from around the world who gather at the United Nations in New York to create a unique ritual for humankind and planet Earth.

Master Atome is an ancestor now—or, as he would say, "The soul is immortal; it never dies." Instead it incarnates, and in each lifetime it leaves behind a body, and only takes with it the lessons learned. Atome's work continues on the higher planes, but his legacy remains vividly present here on Earth.

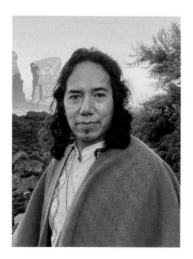

Mindahi Crescencio Bastida Muñoz, Ph.D.

Region: Tultepec, Mexico
Wisdom Tradition: Otomi-Toltec
Organization: The Fountain
Website: The Fountain Earth

Mindahi Crescencio Bastida Muñoz, Ph.D., is the director of the Original Nations Program of The Fountain. He serves as the general coordinator of the Otomi-Toltec Regional Council in Mexico. Bastida's work centers around restoration of the

Original Instructions and ancestral wisdom through the Unification Process based on the Five Earth Mandates. A caretaker of the philosophy and traditions of the Otomi-Toltec peoples, he has been an Otomi-Toltec ritual ceremony officer since 1988. He is a consultant with UNESCO for sacred sites and biocultural issues, and also consults for other United Nations programs.

Bastida has served as a delegate to various commissions and summits on Indigenous rights and sustainability, including the 1992 Earth Summit and the World Summit on Sustainable Development (WSSD, 2002). He was director of the Original Caretakers Program at the Center for Earth Ethics at Union Theological Seminary in New York City between 2015 and 2020 and has been invited to partake in several advisory councils.

He has written on the relation between the state and Indigenous Peoples, intercultural education, collective intellectual property rights and associated traditional knowledge, biocultural sacred sites, and restoration of the Original Instructions through the Unification Process based on the Five Earth Mandates. In Bastida Muñoz's most recent book, *Ancestors: Divine Remembrances of Lineage, Relations and Sacred Sites*, he shares his wisdom on these and other topics.

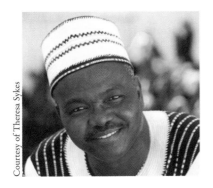

Courtesy of Theresa Sykes

Malidoma Patrice Somé, Ph.D.

Region: Dano, Burkina Faso, West Africa

Wisdom Tradition: Dagara

Organization: Ancestral Events

Malidoma Patrice Somé, Ph.D., West African elder, author and teacher, came to the West as representative of his village in Burkina Faso, West Africa, to share the ancient wisdom and practices that have supported his people for thousands of years. For more than thirty years, Elder Malidoma shared the wisdom of his ancestors and tribal elders: the Dagara Cosmology. He awakened a deep knowing in the hearts and bones of those who recognized in his name, his books, and his voice that the spirit world is inviting the renewal of a deep and abiding relationship with all beings on Earth. Elder Malidoma was the author of several books, including *Ritual: Power, Healing and Community, Of Water and the Spirit: Ritual, Magic and Initiation in the Life of an African Shaman,* and *the Healing Wisdom of Africa: Finding Life Purpose through Nature, Ritual, and Community.* He held three master's degrees and two doctorates from the Sorbonne and Brandeis University. He was an initiated elder in his village in Dano, Burkina Faso. Elder Malidoma became an ancestor in 2021. We honor his powerful spirit and the vast contributions made through his timeless teachings.

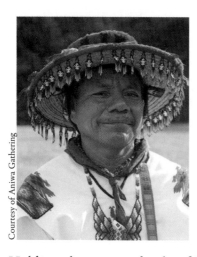

Courtesy of Aniwa Gathering

Modesto Rivera Lemus

Region: Sierra Madre Occidental Mountains, Mexico
Wisdom Tradition: Wixárika (Huichol)
Website: Mexiarts: Magically Handcrafted
Organization: Aniwa Gathering

Modesto Rivera Lemus is an artist, musician, and ritualist of the Wixárika tradition from Nayarit. Holding the esteemed role of Mara'akame, a healer and ceremonial leader, Modesto serves as a conduit, bridging the timeless wisdom of ancient traditions into the contemporary era, and fostering healing and transformation for our planet, humanity, and interpersonal connections.

In the Wirraritari cosmovision, every element, from the fauna that grace the Earth to the spectrum of colors, carries profound symbolism.

Wixárika traditional artworks, employing yarn, beads, and beeswax, are not just visually captivating but also a narrative medium, encapsulating the rich lore and historical tapestry of Modesto's culture. Modesto's artwork is a vibrant testament to Nierika, a sacred space of interconnected realms, and intricately portrays narratives like that of Kauyumari, the Blue Deer, an emblematic spirit intertwined with the psychoactive cactus peyote; or *hikuri*, revered as a sacramental entity in Wixárika culture.

Modesto also shares stories through the *xaweri*, a violin-like instrument integral to Wixárika melodies, often echoing the harmonies of birdsong. Adhering to the path of Wixárika customs, Modesto is an integral part of the Yw'rata community near Tepic, Nayarit, leading pilgrimages to the ancestral homelands of Wirikuta. Modesto is celebrated for his dedication over the last three decades to conserving the Wirraritari cultural legacy. He follows in the footsteps of his father, Eustolio Rivera de la Cruz, a revered Mara'akame, by living his life in nature, hunting and tending to the land.

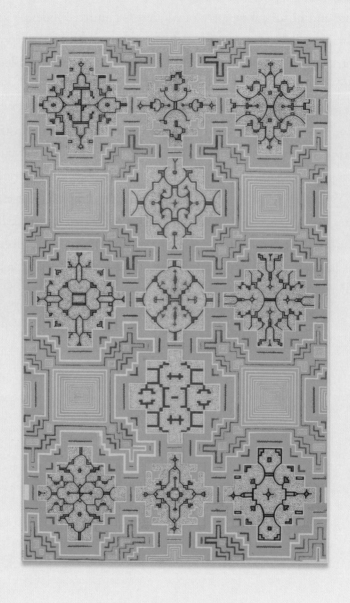

Kené Shipibo Conibo Center
by Sara Flores, Shipibo Traditional Artist

APPENDIX 2

Stewardship

As we conclude this exploration, our journey is far from over. In the forthcoming pages, we will embark on a deeper dive into the underbrush of the Western psychedelic and psychospiritual movement, exploring how we can engage respectfully with spiritual guardians and honor traditional knowledge and nature. I emphasize the significance of reciprocity and maintaining a harmonious connection with Indigenous communities, as this is essential to moving forward in a beneficial way. We can easily become lost or lose what we have all worked hard to contribute to without the proper advisors, as we in the West are still very new to this space. Let's enter this delicate landscape together, exploring diverse perspectives and embracing complexity among the often overlooked, intricate, and sometimes tangled roots of this profound cultural phenomenon. It is a vast topic, so the intention behind what I share is to bring different ideas to the conversation, but in no way is this the only perspective. We must take it all in and move carefully as we build a solid foundation for this work to flourish. Together, we can tap into the transformative potential of psychedelics and plant medicines and wisely move toward a more interconnected, compassionate, and resilient world grounded in mutual trust and mutual benefit. It is our duty to bring this work forward in a way that honors it and those who have walked the path before us.

Spiritual Protocols

While I can't speak for every tradition, based on my experiences and research, it's a practice of respect among Indigenous elders that when they journey to unfamiliar territories, they first seek out the custodians of that land, often the Original People, to request permission for spiritual activities. Upon receiving a blessing, offerings are made to the land, and nothing is taken from it without permission. These offerings serve to honor the land's spiritual guardians and to seek their blessings and protection during the visit. This protocol drastically contrasts with the West's narrative of staking claims to land and taking natural resources and individual rights.

To illustrate the importance of respecting these spiritual protocols, let me share the story of Daniel Northcott, a global adventurer and filmmaker who traveled to forty-two countries over nine years. Each time he went to one of these places, he took home a souvenir. Northcott had accumulated quite a collection on his travels.

One of his explorations found him in a Mayan burial chamber, where he noticed a small, perfectly round object he thought was a stone. His Mayan guide, Gustavo, told him not to take anything and even warned that many had fallen ill or died after doing so, but this item seemed so small and insignificant that he put it in his pocket. Some months later, however, he became sick and learned he had leukemia. When Northcott realized he had broken a sacred law by taking the stone without permission, he tried to find the sacred object to return it, but it was as if it had disappeared. As he neared the end of his life, his family helped him look for it. But it was not found until three years after his death, stored in a collection of shells and stones.

After the artifact resurfaced, the family traveled to the burial chamber with the local guide, who explained that the whole cave system was guarded by mythological spirits called *alux*, pronounced "a-loush." Northcott had taken their toy, one of the balls they played with. Gustavo believed that a curse had been laid upon Northcott, as the ancients warned, which would pass to all his family members until the item was returned. Therefore a ceremony was performed to return the ball to its correct place in the cave.

I know this sounds like something out of an *Indiana Jones* plotline, but Northcott's story is a not a fairy tale, and it reminds me always to stay humble and to respect the spiritual guardians of a place. It is also a story about the repercussions of interfering with the natural order, especially at sacred sites and when engaging in ceremonies.

Throughout this section, we'll discuss some complexities surrounding this topic so you can develop a deeper understanding of how to respectfully engage with these spiritual guardians and ancestral traditions in a way that feels honoring within you. It's a humble learning process and may open your eyes to any blind spots that you may have.

One way to start is by researching the Original Peoples of the land on which you reside, and making sure to honor and acknowledge these ancestors of the land. You can pay your respects to the spiritual guardians of your land, making offerings such as tobacco, water, or fruits. Try sitting on your land and listening to build a relationship with it. Ask the land what it needs from you. Observe the land and its health and well-being. What might it be communicating? Is the ecosystem in balance? How can you provide support?

Reciprocity

When we take something from a place or a community, whether plants, traditions, gold, or water, it's important to give something in return as to not harm that community. *Community* refers to all wildlife, all people, and the ecological biocenosis. I am not implying that these natural resources belong to any one group. Rather, they are part of an intricate, interdependent support system that is stewarded by a people. We also must consider our deepest dedication to the relationships with the people connected in that place and how we nurture and care for them. Practicing reciprocity lets us maintain a right relationship with that community.

The first step is to open up a dialogue. We create reciprocal relationships through an ongoing spiritual exchange, not just a monetary one.

For instance, wild sage has grown quite popular in the spiritual movement. People use it to clear energy and to make sacred space prior to a ceremony. The sage plant is a guardian of the land, but when it is picked from its native land without the proper prayers and cycles of nature, it creates an imbalance in the ecosystem that can leave that land vulnerable. This impacts other plants as well as small animals that use it for cover. In some places, the people of the land where this plant grows in the wild are requesting that the sage be given time to recover from over harvesting. To honor the gift of this medicine, we might consider supporting sustainable sage growers or cultivating our own sage. We can also choose alternatives to sage such as incense, rosemary, or bay leaf. As effective as sage is, so is our intention and presence when performing smoke cleansing rituals.

In 2018 a voice came to me that I called the ancestral heart, a voice that guided me to uplift the voices of ancient wisdom. It requested that I bring the Zulu tribe to Burning Man as a cultural exchange. After receiving three clear signs, I moved forward. It was no easy task taking a group of people to Black Rock City. Rather than creating a formal structure right away, I carefully listened and supported the tribe as specific instructions came from the ancestral heart.

Now years later, the nonprofit Ancestral Heart (named after this ancient voice of wisdom) has helped fund initiatives to support local villages in planting and cultivatng iboga in partnership with Blessings of the Forest, an organization in Gabon founded to preserve the Bwiti biocultural heritage for future generations. Now, we are completing our third land trust in La Sierra Nevada, Colombia, working with the instructions Kogi Kággaba to restore the body of the mother, as the

Mamos say, to allow them to do their sacred work. Giving in this way is so nurturing for the soul. I am so grateful for all that I can give and hope many others can experience this same feeling though their own acts of aligned reciprocity.

The act of reciprocity isn't confined to giving back to Indigenous communities; it also means giving back to organizations that grant people access to plant medicines and psychedelics, as well as organizations that are building infrastructure to help preserve plant medicines for future generations. Further, reciprocity includes supporting policy that ensures the rights of Indigenous communities to protect and rematriate their land and its resources. I've put together a few basic suggestions that may help you begin, below. Remember, reciprocity is not a set formula. It is something you have to choose for yourself by listening and receiving guidance. I only share my process so you may start to connect with your own inner reciprocity process and receive the blessings of it. There are so many ways outside of giving money to show your gratitude to the medicine and its traditions and by promoting respectful use of these practices within your community. Here are a few ways you can give back, to guide your practice of reciprocity:

- Contribute above and beyond the cost or exchange of a medicine or a ceremony, learning traditional knowledge through a class, workshop, or retreat; or receiving a psychedelic therapy session for yourself.
- Give a donation to groups that ensure the ecological or cultural sustainability of a medicine or tradition, or that support ancestral wisdom keepers.
- Make a donation or offering every time you notice the medicine or traditional knowledge is working in your life and blessing you. This is unlimited because the blessings always continue to flow, but I have seen that gift become more potent when reciprocity is added.

- Make regular, consistent donations of money or your time to support groups, advocacy groups, legal policy initiatives, or community initiatives that support wisdom keepers and also marginalized groups.

In these ways, you can pay it forward for the medicine so it may support people, both now and in future generations. It's also important to note that many Indigenous communities have been disrupted by Western influence, and deep relationships of reciprocity take many years to establish. It's important to honor the sacredness of Indigenous communities by refraining from visiting unless you've received a formal invitation and are willing to abide by their spiritual protocols. Unfortunately, some retreats and tours, while perhaps well-intentioned, inadvertently contribute to the erosion of these original cultures. Let's prioritize safeguarding the original ways of life by being mindful of our actions and ensuring we do not inadvertently do harm.

Distinguishing between ceremonies conducted with integrity and cultural respect versus those lacking such qualities involves research, interviewing individuals who are part of the community, and one's ability to ask relevant questions to the facilitator or traditional practitioner. These ceremonies typically serve spiritual or cultural purposes, emphasizing inclusivity and collaboration with the traditional community. If the facilitator is not from the tradition's lineage , ask where they have trained, for how long, and if they have been given the blessing to conduct this type of ceremony. Many times, these types of ceremonies require adherence to specific protocols outlined by the tradition. Be wary of ceremonies that trivialize cultural protocols, or lack a meaningful link to original wisdom keepers of the traditions. By attentively assessing factors such as authenticity, purpose, inclusivity, and community involvement, individuals can better discern whether a ceremony upholds principles of respect and integrity toward traditional cultures.

Cultural Appreciation

Cultural appreciation is a term I propose to encourage a more compassionate and respectful approach to engaging with ancient lineages, as opposed to the problematic *cultural mining*, or *cultural appropriation*. As Westerners, we have the privilege of encountering cultural artifacts and practices from various societies, so we must treat them with the reverence they deserve.

When we are influenced by elements from other cultures, we should do so authentically and respectfully. For example, ceremonial headdresses that are worn by the Yawanawá in the Amazon or the Comanche war bonnets made of Eagle feathers are symbols of honor, earned through exceptional acts of service. These headdresses should only be worn by those who have received them through proper rites or ceremonies (in some traditions they are only presented to men). Tribal regalia are not costumes, and wearing them outside their intended context devalues their historical and cultural significance.

This concept of cultural appreciation extends to the realm of psychedelic medicines. As the field of psychedelic therapy advances, it is essential that large corporations acknowledge Indigenous wisdom and the hard work of the underground psychedelic movement. I'm excited by the possibility of a refocus on fostering collective learning and respecting the thousands of years of knowledge held by Indigenous cultures.

A decade ago, the Indigenous people of the Amazon Forest called for a halt to corporations exploiting their medicines for profit, highlighting the need for Indigenous peoples worldwide to stand together as guardians of the planet. It's also vital for corporations to share their scientific discoveries and make therapeutic treatments and training accessible to Indigenous communities.

Companies such as Journey Colab and Woven Science have developed comprehensive reciprocity models that take a respectful approach to engaging with Indigenous wisdom. Such models should guide the entire corporate, for-profit psychedelic space, helping to prevent acts of biopiracy and promoting a more compassionate and inclusive future.

Within the framework established by the United Nations, UNESCO, and the Nagoya Protocol, there exist legal mechanisms designed to safeguard the biocultural and traditional knowledge linked to plant medicines. Particularly significant is the provision within the Nagoya Protocol which prohibits the patenting of genetic resources, including alkaloids like ibogaine, if they are part of biocultural traditional knowledge without prior consent and benefit-sharing agreements. Noteworthy achievements include the groundbreaking agreement reached with the San and Khoi peoples of South Africa regarding reciprocity concerning the traditional knowledge surrounding rooibos tea. Companies holding illegal patents of biocultural knowledge could potentially face substantial penalties in the future. The return of cultural sacred objects to Indigenous peoples from museums, along with evolving legal protections and the increasing number of cases supporting Indigenous claims, underscore the importance for companies to consider these regulations and start working alongside keepers of biocultural knowledge. Many indigenous groups, including the Bwiti, are in the process of registering their biocultural claims with UNESCO to demonstrate a clear statement: there are many eyes paying attention and actions will be taken against organizations that do not respect these sanctions.

Deeper Understanding

In reaction to the Western psychedelic movement and current ecological crisis, the International Council of Thirteen Indigenous Grandmothers formed a global alliance of Indigenous keepers of sacred wisdom as a collective voice for the Earth, protection of ancient traditions, and elder wisdom. Since 2004, they have been letting the world know where they stand concerning their roles as guardians of nature and the planet.

Tribes in the Amazon along with other Indigenous nations globally unified to declare, "We were here before governments came, and we will be here after governments leave." They advocate against unauthorized exploitation of their forest resources and traditional medicines, emphasizing the importance of respectful usage accompanied by the original teachings. Calling upon First Nations peoples worldwide to assert their inherent responsibility as custodians of the Earth, they advocate for solidarity in reclaiming their birthright as planetary stewards.

In contrast to the ceremonial use of these plant medicines practiced by the lineage keepers, they're often used casually outside of their original context. One example is the popularization of microdosing, or taking a psychoactive plant in a sub-perceptual dose, specifically in the context of "enhancing performance," or taking them like a nutritional supplement rather than using them for the deeper spiritual healing that comes from intentional use, or as a tool for contemplative work. The use of intentions and prayer, and often with the guidance of a traditional practitioner, plays a role in supporting the experience and its effects. When we reduce the practice, we lose the respect of something sacred, and it devalues it and our own appreciation for this gift.

This reductionist concept can also be seen in novices who proclaim themselves *facilitators* or *sitters*, someone who supports an individual or group experience with plant medicine or psychedelics without any formal training, initiation from a lineage or apprenticeship from a long-time practitioner. Often, they lack a basic understanding of trauma or mental health. These self-appointed healers or facilitators are akin to individuals impersonating doctors without the required training and qualifications. Unfortunately, their misguided efforts can lead to serious consequences, including mental instability, psychosis, injury, or even loss of life.

Iboga, as many know in the West, has safety risks and there are spiritual technologies and rituals within the cosmology and tradition of Bwiti that ensure the initiate's safe passage. In Gabon, mastering the traditional knowledge system of the Bwiti takes ten and sometimes up to twenty-five years depending on the initiate. Part of the reason for this lengthy apprenticeship is understanding these protocols that create a safe and effective initiation. In some traditions, specific formats and rituals have been given to initiates for work with iboga that were created to address the nuances of the Western psyche. Different rites are performed for each individual, depending on divination or their place within their spiritual path, for instance, rituals for males to help them understand the initiation of manhood. Often a person will not receive information or teachings until he has completed various levels of his initiation. Just as a flower cannot fully bloom until it first forms into a bud, no steps can be bypassed.

When I started working at Crossroads, I had a team of doctors and nurses alongside me. My job was preparing the person for the ceremony, providing the ceremonial elements in a clinical setting and supporting the integration. Even on the third day when I gave 5-MeO-DMT to the participants, I had a nurse or doctor alongside me.

As a started my own work, my partner, a psychologist, was often alongside me and we processed the sessions and retreats together afterward. Several years later, when I got the blessing to provide healing work with iboga, I was told that I could offer psychospiritual healing with iboga. But, I was told, I was not a nima, so I could not call those healings Bwiti initiations, like the ones performed by nima in Gabon. I was told that I still needed to continue my training and I had not "graduated". In Gabon, I was also told that if I wanted to be a nima and to give initiations that I had to move there and fully dedicate myself to study. There may be a chance, as I continue to go to Gabon and grow in my practice of Bwiti, that I could be a nima, but even with a decade of experience, it could take another ten years, or more—who can say for sure? I don't have any goals or attachment to any titles, just a devotion to the practice of Bwiti. The knowledge system of Bwiti is one of the most complex and vast, and one must know it to be nima.

When Gabon closed its borders to outside visitors, Joseph and I started doing regular Zoom calls with our Bwiti families to receive teachings and stay connected. I asked one of my Missoko elders, "Is it practical for Westerners to become nima?" His response felt designed to spur contemplation on the context, "First you would need a *mousingi,* the skin of a small spotted creature that looks like a serval, to do your spiritual works, and a nima also wears the skin of a panther (in Missoko). I don't know if there are enough panther in the jungle for all the Westerners that would want to be nima." I am aware that this is not the practice in all traditions, but I can say great sacrifices must be made for one to be passed the power. When one becomes nima, they are literally given a transference of the power of the lineage held in an energy transmission from nima to nima and in sacred objects that contain this power. It is a huge responsibility.

These potent medicines, like iboga, are bridges to the spiritual domain, to be shared among all as a gift or treasure for humanity. However it's crucial to recognize the established protocols endorsed by genuine wisdom keepers, as they serve the safety of all involved, including practitioners. I convey these thoughts with compassion, acknowledging that numerous unfortunate or tragic occurrences can be averted through the implementation of proper infrastructure that honors the wisdom of Indigenous elders and incorporates the harm reduction and educational practices they have cultivated over centuries.

The Path to Legalization

Contemporary psychedelic therapy has come a long way from the unregulated and uninformed psychedelic first wave. Structured protocols, therapeutic frameworks, and harm reduction practices to mitigate risks and optimize therapeutic potential have been developed. The Multidisciplinary Association for Psychedelic Studies (MAPS) offers a psychedelic training program with unique benefits. Its peer review aspect, for instance, allows aspiring psychedelic therapists to receive feedback from experienced practitioners, thus helping to identify areas for improvement and foster professional growth. A combination of theoretical knowledge, practical experience, and guidance from experienced mentors is the best way to become a proficient facilitator or psychedelic therapist. The framework, as laid out by Annie and Michael Mithofer, involves a therapy pair, typically male and female. This cofacilitation approach definitely fills some gaps in experience that might occur with one newly training therapist. But there is still a long way to go, as the path to masterful facilitation is a lifelong process, and one must approach the journey with humility, opening oneself to continued education, self-reflection, and a commitment to refining one's skills. Experience with mystical experiences and altered states is also required, as one cannot support navigating these sometimes intense experiences without thoroughly knowing the terrain themselves.

In envisioning the integration of psychedelics and plant medicines into our society, it's imperative to establish transparent and responsible pathways, rooted in careful and informed practices. However, we must critically assess: have we taken sufficient steps?

In my view, extending the training requirements for practitioners, particularly therapists, should be a priority. This extension should include an emphasis on ethics education, peer review processes, apprenticeships, and thorough background checks. Additionally, basic first aid training and CPR certification should be mandatory for all involved. Moreover, personal experience with altered states of consciousness is a foundational prerequisite for anyone engaging in this field. Yet individual training is only part of the equation; nurturing a supportive community is equally essential.

Currently, our educational landscape often perpetuates outdated narratives surrounding the war on drugs, such as those propagated by programs like Drug Abuse Resistance Education (D.A.R.E.) in high schools. If we're inundating media with information about psychedelics and plant medicines, we must also address the impact on youth and prioritize harm reduction. Take, for example, the case of ketamine, heralded as a treatment for depression. Its medicinal use has inadvertently fueled illegal market activities and recreational consumption, leading to tragic consequences such as deaths resulting from street ketamine laced other substances including fentanyl. Youth, lacking legal access routes, are particularly vulnerable to the risks associated with the resurgence of psychedelics. Thus we must diligently consider strategies to safeguard them from harm.

In areas where our knowledge of these medicines spans mere decades rather than centuries, developing a robust framework to support the integration of the psychedelic movement could pave the way for legalization as the natural next step in the evolution of this process.

Purification

Many traditions begin their ceremonies with days of purification before participants undergo an initiatory ritual or ingest any psychoactive plants or sacraments. Some rites or customs require preparatory cleansing of the body, sometimes with purgatory plants that are ingested to induce vomiting. In the Bwiti tradition, one goes through a series of spiritual baths made with cleansing plants and clays. These rituals, performed by traditional Bwiti healers, may also include thorough confessions made by the initiate intended to make peace with self-criticism, being dishonest to ourselves or others, withholding something we feel we need to say, or harm we have done to others.

Deep in the jungles of South America, in curanderismo traditions, as discussed in chapter 9, dietas are a form of purification used to allow one's communication with plants and can take anywhere from several weeks to a year. These dietas involve working with a specific plant that the traditional medicine practitioner chooses based on the individual's needs, using ayahuasca as the intermediary to open plant communication. An aspect of the dieta is to open our awareness with respect to our relationship with normal desires by eliminating salt, spice, alcohol, sex, fats, and sweets. The primary purpose being to cultivate a relationship with the subtle soul of the plant to understand its role within the cosmology of the plant kingdom and spiritual realms; the elimination opens the line of communication.

These dietas and other purification protocols also can help people open themselves to the sensitivities necessary to work as a traditional practitioner, allowing the plants to work through them to inform their understanding of the healing arts. Typically, one does not take a dieta for that reason, to serve medicine to others, but the path starts to become clear over time with the guidance of a traditional elder of the lineage—sometimes as a complete surprise to the individual.

My own experiences in engaging with purification rituals, for myself and others, have shown me that these rituals increase the depth of the work and support the medicine in its process. The greater the sincerity of the individual entering purification, the more power the medicine has to transform them. This is why it is advised to start agenda-free. As I see it, without purification, the medicine has to do a lot of heavy lifting to cleanse the person, which limits its ability to accomplish the deeper mystical work.

Cultural Authenticity

During my time with the Kogi Kággaba, when they spoke of ancestral knowledge I would notice the mamos pause and ask the spirits' permission to share something. Sometimes after asking, the mamo would say, "I am sorry; I cannot share this information." Historically, nearly every initiatic tradition, ancestral lineage, or mystery school contained levels of secrecy, as what is sacred must remain behind some level of a veil to the uninitiated. Some traditions even believed you would be punished or have your power stripped if you revealed the secrets to non-adepts.

Malidoma Patrice Somé shared that in the Dagara tradition, the spirits know when you have broken your pact and the retribution often times comes swiftly. If such sacred information is used in sloppy or misguided ways, it won't produce the same results. The real recipe always lives in the heart of the practitioner. Several times in receiving teachings from Māori elders, our group was given specific protocols or prayers, but we were told not to teach these techniques to others; they were given to us for our personal healing only.

In contrast, in Western culture, once someone learns something, they are often eager to share it on social media even before they have embodied it. Sacred knowledge is protected for this very reason. This is not just about authenticity; it is a safeguard to shield the ancients' wisdom from being distorted or taken out of context. Those tricky egos love to inflate around the accumulation of knowledge and achievement, and can it be so subtle that it goes unnoticed and is difficult to weed out once it has taken root. Engaging with a mentor consistently and being part of an authentic and empathetic community empowers individuals to express themselves with courage, sincerity, integrity, and authenticity. It is wise to tread with humility and receptivity, understanding that we cannot take for granted the use of traditional wisdom without proper reverence and respect. Power is not in the knowing or the showing; it is in the being. You can only truly learn from those who embody the wisdom; likewise, you can't teach anything in a useful way without embodying it yourself. You become the light that acts as a lantern for others through your authentic expression of self.

In this spirit, I encourage you to draw inspiration from ancient knowledge systems and expand your awareness of our vast cosmos. Perhaps you could begin by exploring the veins of your own ancestral culture and uncovering your unique connection to your forebears. I believe that every soul has left a trail of breadcrumbs leading back to their most authentic self.

In my case, my Great-Great-Grandmother Jesus, an open-hearted widow, ran a boarding house, providing shelter for migrant laborers so she could provide for two daughters as a single mother. It is through this diverse upbringing that my family integrated elements of Afro-Mestizo spirituality into our traditions. My great-great-grandmother, whose background was Oaxacan mestiza (Mixtec, Triqui, and Mexica) practiced a blend of Santeria and mystical Catholicism, which was introduced to the region around four hundred years ago by Africa, slaves brought by Spanish colonists. Following Mexico's liberation from Spain, slavery was abolished, and African Americans migrated from the United States via the underground railroad in the early 1800s. Oaxaca stands out as one of Mexico's most culturally diverse regions, home to sixteen distinct indigenous groups. For several generations, as that is as far as I could dig back, my mother line has practiced this blend of ethnic traditions, rooted in ceremonial rituals, healing, prayer, and divination.

My grandfather, Richard Ortega, was the last person in the family to practice. He called himself Catholic but I sense that was because living in America, he could only practice in Catholic churches. I remember his devotion. He never missed a mass, no matter what city he was in. My mother said he still held his beliefs from his unconventional animist upbringing. As I traced my ancestors' spiritual practice, I discovered the connection to equatorial African Yoruba traditions, which have stark similarities to Bwiti. I still get goose bumps to think that it was in my ancestral homelands of Mexico that I got invited to work at Crossroads, which led me down a path of reclaiming my families Afro-Mestiza mystical practices.

While my other lineage connections on my father's side are less clear, my grandma Hazel grew up in Calgary, Canada. She was mostly of European descent and as a child was put in an orphanage with her four brothers and sisters after their mother died. They hopped a train, like the kids in *The Boxcar Children*, after escaping the orphanage and landed in Spokane, Washington. Hazel and her identical twin sister

Pearl married brothers and they each had many children, one of whom Patricia, gave birth to my father. She was addicted to pills and Hazel came over to see my papa as a newborn, laying in a crib, skinny and wearing a soiled diaper. Hazel said to Patricia, this baby doesn't look too good. And Patricia replied, "do you want to take him?" So Hazel adopted him as an infant.

Hazel was one the matriarchs of our family, akin to the grandmother killer whales that lead their pods and teach the family how to survive and thrive. She took my mother under her wing; she was just eighteen when she had me. My mother's mother, also named Patricia, died of cancer at age 42 just weeks before I was born. Hazel taught my mother how to be a mother, and she didn't just pass down parenting skills, but also a deep reverence for nature, caring, and spirituality.

However both lineages also bore a massive debt of ancestral trauma. The untimely deaths and hardships within the family, addiction, and the shadow of shame that lingered through generations reflect the darker undercurrents of our family history. Like the diverse pods of killer whales throughout the world, each adapting to unique environments and challenges, the matriarchy in my family too had its set of original principles for survival which my grandmother and mother passed to me. The trauma carried by the men in our lineage contrasted sharply with the resilience and overcoming spirit of many of the women of my lineage. During my younger years, I struggled to come to terms with the lack of support from the masculine. But this realization brought me into a deep reverence and respect for the many initiations my family had endured and helped me to transmute the trauma through the power of the original principles of the matriarchal lineage carried through the bloodline.

Exchange

When it comes to exchanging money for initiatory work, not every culture believes in giving away healing for free or almost free. This "oath of poverty" originated in the Judeo-Christian worldview and in some Eastern traditions such as Buddhism and Taoist beliefs. But in reality, it is not sustainable to work this way unless spiritual healers are part of an infrastructure that collects a regular tithe from the people it serves. I have never met a tribe or traditional medicine man or woman with health insurance or much in the way of reserves to help them in a catastrophe, or who didn't need support to maintain the space where they host healing ceremonies. Bayo Akomolafe, the Yoruba speaker and author, shares another narrative around financial exchanges:

> Where I come from, the sacred is irretrievably entangled with harvesting good yams, prosperity, and consulting the rainmaker. Eating well, supporting one's community, and being compensated for offering oneself to a process are matters of the economy—and economics is always caught up in larger unfinished questions about what it means to be a subject of modern civilization, what it means to be with others in the community, what material commitments we make to the networks of suffering around us.

It is a commonplace to pay what some might consider a high price for initiations with the Bwiti, ranging from $1,000 to $4,500. These initiations take a lot of preparation and staging. Throughout the initiation, there will be harpists and other healers who will expect gifts from you as well, to recognize their role in the initiation. So, many times, the final level of contribution to the village can be much more than the initial cost discussed, as a blessing is expected to recognize the people who showed up and contributed on your behalf. And in what other way could we convey this work's immeasurable value besides financial exchange?

One of my friends, the Colombian medicine man Gustavo Fernandez, says his elders taught him that giving should hurt, and if it doesn't, you should give more. That means if you have a lot, your giving should reflect the value of the healing you receive, in scale to what you have. Giving a little can hurt if you are not in a good financial position. Yet suppose you are a billionaire, and you took the San Pedro medicine and developed a profound creative idea that greatly contributed to creating that wealth. In that case, a fair exchange might look like giving a portion of the profits as a form of reciprocity. Some members of tribes I've worked with in Gabon will ask the spirits how much an initiate should pay, and whatever answer they receive through divination, that is the price. One person might be asked to give €550, and another might be told to give €5,000. At my third Bwiti initiation, I was asked to pay more than my partner. There was no explanation for why; that was just how it was.

I also feel a bit uneasy about individuals who profit through investment in psychedelic companies, only to pocket enormous sums for themselves rather than supporting the infrastructure or individuals who do the work. It's diverting resources from the people serving the medicine, and from the organizations that support the Indigenous wisdom keepers of these traditions. I believe these profits need to go into feeding the movement by funding centers for healing—beautiful sacred medicine sanctuaries that can be preserved for retreats, and programs accessible to those underserved in the space.

If we put resources into enriching the Original Peoples and their communities, this would help them preserve invaluable cultural wisdom and would support continued accessibility for all people. This is an essential and often missing piece that must be considered for this movement to flourish adequately and equitably.

Access

If you have access to healing medicine, it's a blessing. This also means being mindful of how often you are taking medicines such as ayahuasca or iboga. Although there are many ways to work with ayahuasca, the way that I am most familiar with involves following a special diet while in isolation, so the plants can do their deepest work. In some initiatic traditions, people only receive the sacrament one time. In Bwiti, the initiatic process is designed for a deep reset and the integration period typically lasts for about a year. You don't need to keep taking the medicine unless you are on a specific path where it is required, such as the path of becoming a nima or initiator. And in the past select few received it; those individuals came of their own accord. They found the hidden path because they were ripe to find it. No one had to clear the path for them.

In my experience, I have never seen any sincere, ready person fail to find a way or the resources. On the other hand, some people are enabled to take the medicine too soon and have very rough journeys and integration experiences. I observed this while working at the ibogaine clinic when family members would send a loved one to do ibogaine to cure their opiate addiction. Many times it gave them a chance they wouldn't have had, but some weren't invested in doing the work necessary to stay sober. You have to have some skin in the game to be invested in the hard work required to make treatment successful. Each person must engage with the path they find and be curious about their barriers because there is nearly always a way. This process of how the path opens for you and its timing is part of the journey.

The truth is that highly traumatized individuals are not always the best candidates for this work. In addition, some of these individuals come from communities with underlying social and economic problems, and once they return home, those troubles they had escaped from with drugs become more painfully present. We have some major societal issues that we all need to face collectively and part of that is putting the net in place to hold those who are vulnerable during their healing process. We cannot rush the process of setting the foundation necessary for responsible psychedelic and plant medicine stewardship and use. Proper stewardship requires time to create infrastructure and train qualified facilitators who can provide effective and meaningful outcomes.

Abuses of Power

The topic of abuse of power in the psychedelic community could be a book in itself. To preface what I have to say here, I've had several teachers, whom I later learned had compromised their integrity in some way. Many of these abuses of power were of a sexual nature, and from my experience in Bwiti and Mesoamerican traditions, this is not uncommon. I was not personally involved in the incidents, so it's not my place to publicly call them out. Situations like these should be addressed within the communities affected. What I will say is, this is where it is key to have personal and reputable referrals for any kind of psychedelic or plant medicine work that you do.

One thing that is very clear in my mind is that once you have entered into a healing relationship with someone, especially with psychoactive substances that distort perception, you should not be engaging in any kind of romantic relationship with that person. In Bwiti initiations, for example, your adepts are considered your children, and of course one should not be sexual with their children. The Association of State and Provincial Psychology Boards and American Psychological Association ethics exams clearly state how many years must pass before one can consider having a relationship with a former patient. Although the limits may differ slightly from state to state, the penalty for not adhering to this rule is the loss of one's psychologist license to practice. And this is without involving any psychedelics, which adds other layers of complexity to the situation.

The best way to avoid being in a compromised position is to work with facilitators who adhere to strict ethical guidelines. Make sure your facilitator can be vouched for by someone who knows their work well. The more character references you can gather, the better. Once you take the medicine, you cannot know what will happen. I recall a story of some women who went to a village in the Amazon and sat in ceremony with a convicted sex offender. Several of the women were molested by this person during the ceremony, and the curanderos did nothing about it. A foundational principle of working with psychedelics and plant medicines is "set and setting"—so make sure your setting is safe. If you're uncertain, don't do it. There are plenty of legal plant medicine retreat centers internationally that are doing reputable work.

Sadly, money abuses among tribal leaders are also common. Many of these cultures have been infiltrated by Western materialism. Although not always the case, I have personally seen tribal leaders misappropriate funds for lavish vacations and luxury goods like Louis Vuitton bags. Supporting nonprofit organizations and project-based initiatives rather than just sending money to a village can be an effective way to avoid misuse of funds.

The bigger issue within the psychedelic movement is that we must urgently establish protocols for how to address bad actors calling themselves facilitators. How do we in the movement prevent such questionable guides from creating more harm? While acknowledging the complexity of this issue, we can initiate progress by cultivating accountability within the psychedelic community through fostering of open dialogue and developing feedback mechanisms. By establishing community-led initiatives aimed at addressing instances of misconduct or unethical behavior among facilitators, we can prioritize restorative approaches when appropriate. Additionally, empowering participants to advocate for their own well-being is crucial; this can be achieved by providing comprehensive information on their rights, informed consent procedures, and accessible channels for reporting concerns. Emphasizing transparent communication between facilitators and participants throughout the therapeutic journey further strengthens the integrity of the process.

Sustainability

Due to the rapid growth in the use of psychedelic plants for healing and psychospiritual ceremonial use, these plants are becoming increasingly threatened, as Western culture does not realize how ecologically sensitive and endangered they are. Iboga, peyote, and the bufotoxin of the *Incilius alvarius* toad are Earth medicines deeply connected to the sacred lands of native peoples. They are part of complex ecosystems. For example, the *Tabernanthe iboga* plant is related to the okoume trees. The elephants pull on the shrub when picking the fruits, adding strength to the iboga plants' roots. And the mycorrhizal network deep in the jungle soils influences the development of the thirty known alkaloids in this plant. By respecting these endangered plants, we can sustain their presence for generations.

It is important to remember that most, if not all, Indigenous tribes have been taken advantage of by corporations that have repeatedly tried to obtain rights to drill oil or extract minerals from sacred lands. As a result, asking questions, even coming from a supportive place, can be seen as taking time and, in effect, resources. It is crucial to consider reciprocity and cultural sensitivity. Please support organizations such as the International Center for Ethnobotanical Education, Research and Service (ICEERS), Blessings of the Forest, Chacruna Institute for Psychedelic Plant Medicines, or my organization, Ancestral Heart, all of which are well established and are educated in the intricate cultural sensitivities required to support and maintain these relationships.

Another primary concern of the psychedelic movement is that most pharmaceutical synthetic drugs, including ketamine, are manufactured using fossil fuels. The petroleum pharmaceutical manufacturing process has been used since 1907 and is responsible for up to ninety-nine percent of these drugs. However other solvents could be substituted, sourced from nonpetroleum sources. Alternatives are now being researched to replace petroleum in the pharmaceutical feedstocks and reagents—from plant-based alternatives like pineapples to electrochemical activation.

Why is this relevant to our conversation here? Integration and interconnection are the foundations of psychedelic healing. These concepts must be woven into all aspects of the psychedelic space, from our personal lives to the global network at play in the use of psychedelics. Integration ultimately includes us finding a harmonious relationship with nature.

Another sustainable alternative to these delicate medicines is the psilocybin mushroom, which grows rapidly and is far more widely available. Researchers are also investigating novel methods of producing synthetic psychedelic compounds, such as alternative reagents and fermentation processes, which could potentially offer more sustainable options compared to petroleum-based methods of pharmaceutical manufacturing. The media needs to be educated to ensure they communicate these critical issues to the public.

Media, Influencers, and Psychedelics

Increasingly, celebrities, influencers, and mainstream media are becoming more vocal in the psychedelic space. The duty of care includes the responsibility of doing research and seeking expert advice on how to approach the topic. The publicity may cause surges in demand and bring psychedelic tourism that could have negative cultural impacts on small indigenous communities. Influencers have a great opportunity and duty to amplify the voices of Indigenous leaders, activists, and communities. By providing a platform for Indigenous perspectives, they can raise awareness about Indigenous rights, cultural heritage, and environmental stewardship. Influencers should encourage and caution, advocating for responsible and respectful practices in engaging with indigenous traditions and plant medicines. They can educate their audience about the importance of cultural sensitivity, environmental conservation, and supporting local communities.

As someone who has participated in podcasts, spoken at conferences, been interviewed for news channels, featured in numerous articles on psychedelics, and authored a book on the topic, I, too, have contributed to this promotion. My goal is not to stifle crucial discussions but to urge individuals with influence to educate themselves and take responsibility for their impact when discussing psychedelics and plant medicines.

Plant Medicines

Iboga

Iboga is a plant native to the jungles of Gabon, a small country about the size of the state of Colorado, located on the west coast of Equatorial Africa. Recent studies indicate that iboga's root bark contains between thirty and eighty unique alkaloids, a remarkable level of biodiversity influenced by factors such as subspecies and the plant's age. Root bark shavings containing medicinal properties are extracted from the inner layer of the root at seven years (when cultivated) and can be fifty years or older if found in the wild. The complexity not only contributes to the therapeutic potential but also underscores the significance as one of nature's most intricate and fascinating botanical specimens. Iboga is not a traditional psychedelic; instead, it is categorized as an oneirophrenic, attributed to the dreamlike nature of the visions it produces when ingested.

The most prevalent alkaloid derived from iboga, and known in the West, is ibogaine. Ibogaine is what is known as an addiction interrupter, meaning that upon ingesting a flood dose, which is done only in a medically supervised environment, the alkaloid works specifically on the kappa opioid receptor to "reset" it, thus allowing someone physically addicted to opiates to come out of the session without any opiate withdrawal symptoms or cravings.

On a surface level, ibogaine seems like a profound answer for treating addiction. From a phenomenological perspective, looking more deeply at the experiences people have with it, they often go through a life review that can address events and traumas in their early years, providing insights that allow the journeyer to integrate the knowledge and move forward from substance dependency.

This plant has recently gained popularity as an substance use disorder treatment in Western culture. As a result of the increased demand for iboga and over-harvesting of the "holy wood" by poachers to sell on the illegal market in the West, the two hundred villages that are left practicing Bwiti and the initiatory rites of passage are under threat.

While it holds promise for addressing the opioid crisis, the iboga plant takes at least seven years to grow before the alkaloids mature and the root bark can be harvested for use in ceremonies. This plant is sensitive to the environment in which it's cultivated. Iboga has only been known to grow near sea level, specifically in soil conditions only found within Earth's equatorial jungles. Some Bwiti elders dispute its ability to thrive outside of equatorial regions, due to the fragility of seeds in transport.

Iboga is a plant legally protected by the Gabonese government and the United National sanctions under the Nagoya Protocol. Its significance goes beyond its therapeutic benefits, as it has been deemed a cultural treasure of Gabon. Shipping iboga outside Gabon is strictly illegal as of February 2019. Those caught attempting to export it may face severe consequences, including fines or imprisonment. Unfortunately, the illegal market for *Tabernanthe iboga* is fueled by cartel-like groups, contributing to crime and the destruction of precious ecosystems. We need to be cautious of any legislation passed with no mention of reciprocity or honoring the Nagoya Protocol. Gabon was the first country to sign this supplementary agreement to the Convention of Biodiversity. This demonstrates Gabonese and Bwiti desire to protect their cultural heritage, which must be acknowledged and supported.

Blessings of the Forest is a Gabonese nonprofit organization working with local Bwiti villages to support the cultivation of sustainable iboga and preserve the ancestral tradition of Bwiti to ensure the future of this sacred medicine. Individuals are encouraged to support grass roots organizations like Blessings of the Forest if they participate in any ceremony or have in the past, to offset the cultural impacts of Westerners visiting Gabon and using iboga in traditional ceremonies.

At present, due to the lack of availability of the plant iboga, ibogaine is being made by semi-synthetic means, using a plant that is more environmentally sustainable called *Voacanga africana*. Producing ibogaine from alternate sources like *Voacanga africana*—which is what most ibogaine clinics use, and which DemeRx is advancing through the FDA—will reduce negative impact and pressure on wild plant populations in Gabon and Central Africa. Companies are now working on processes to fully synthesize ibogaine, but they haven't determined how to make it on a larger scale at this time. Most international ibogaine clinics are not using ibogaine from iboga, but unfortunately many of them operate in a legal grey area and some still do.

Having pharmaceutical grade ibogaine for clinical use could make therapies easier to access, yet we also have to consider ethical and sustainability issues. Iboga or its derivative, ibogaine, should never be taken alone, or with an inexperienced guide. These substances pose significant medical risks and can lead to cardiac issues and temporary psychosis. Iboga is a QT prolonger, affecting the intervals of the heart's rhythm. Even microdosing can be fatal for individuals with pre-existing QT prolongation or abnormalities. I have seen the most advanced psychonauts as well as uninitiated facilitators put themselves or others in the hospital—and they are fortunate to be alive. Others have not been so lucky.

Choosing to work with ibogaine or iboga is a serious decision. Make sure to educate yourself, and work with facilitators who adhere to proper safety protocols and who understand the complexities of this medicine. In Gabon, Bwiti nima initiates train for at least ten years before they are entrusted with serving the plant. Medical expertise and apprenticeships are needed to fully grasp the responsibilities associated with iboga and ibogaine. I have a doctor who looks at every EKG from potential retreat participants to ensure they are safe to participate. Be especially wary of practitioners who do not follow proper safety protocols or who don't take safety seriously enough. And whatever you do, please don't buy iboga on the illegal market, including Facebook and Instagram.

I am grateful to the ibogaine community for establishing safety standards and screening protocols, which make ingesting iboga incredibly safe when done correctly in a medically supervised setting.

Above all else, we must honor the cultural and natural heritage of Gabon by approaching *Tabernanthe iboga* with caution and respect. We need to preserve its wisdom and protect the fragile communities and ecosystems intertwined with its existence.

Peyote

Peyote is a cactus native to regions of Texas and Mexico. It is used as a sacrament in the traditions of Native American tribes like the Lakota Sioux and Comanche, and by the Original People of Mexico and Mēxica or Nahuas, as well as the Wixárika, also known as the Huichol. The Wixárika hold a place in the central Mexican mountains as sacred. They believe this location was the birthplace of peyote, called *hikuri,* the spirit of the Blue Deer in their tradition. Today, the Wixárika have been driven off much of their homelands with little access to resources, and the land they inhabit is difficult to cultivate food on.

Every year a pilgrimage takes place to Wirikuta, where people hike through the mountains on a journey to harvest the sacred peyote buttons for ceremony. But this cherished area has been purchased by mining companies and private landowners, which makes the pilgrimage more difficult every year. Over the last decade, mining has been destroying the sacred lands and much of the peyote that has grown there for centuries. It's important to note that a single peyote button can take up to thirteen years to mature, adding to the increasing concerns for the protection of the Wixárika biocultural heritage.

Many American Indigenous nations have expressed concern with the psychedelic movement's impact on the illegal harvesting of peyote. Many tribes have been given special permission to do prayers and ceremonies with peyote under the Religious Freedom Act, and they have concerns that the peyote will be depleted if it is included in decriminalization legislation. A statement was issued by the National Council of Native American Churches and the Indigenous Peyote Conservation Initiative, founded to address the sensitivity of this plant and help preserve traditions that use it. The decriminalization movement did honor the Native American Churches' request, but other threatened plants, such as iboga, need to be included as sensitive plants.

As an alternative to peyote, currently the San Pedro cactus thrives in vast numbers across the southwestern United States. It contains mescaline, the same psychedelic alkaloid found in peyote. Synthetic mescaline is also widely available. We can further support tribes that use peyote by returning wild harvested plants kept in captivity to help restore the cultivation of this sacred species.

5-MeO-DMT from the Sonoran Desert Toad

The Sonoran Desert toad (Incilius alvarius) secretes a bufotoxin containing 5-MeO-DMT, a potent psychoactive tryptamine. While Iconography in ancient Mesoamerican artifacts and temples potentially allude to historical use, there's no definitive record of traditional Indigenous practices involving this substance. Extracting the venom, while not typically fatal to the toad, leaves it vulnerable to predators.

When vaporized and inhaled, the 5-MeO-DMT from the Sonoran Desert toad's secretion rapidly induces profound changes in brain activity categorized by EEG as a high-gamma frequency state. This electrical pattern is associated with subjective experiences of oneness or nonduality, mirroring states of consciousness typically achieved only through extensive meditation practice.

Recent years have seen a surge in mainstream interest fueled by

272 ⊙ Appendix 2

celebrity endorsements and media coverage. While potentially well-intentioned, this attention has led to increased psychedelic tourism and environmental strain on the toad's delicate desert habitat. As well, media portrayals gloss over the intensity of preparation and integration required for using this potent medicine that, as Tim Ferriss and Michael Pollan both have shared, is not a fit for everyone.

Local tribes, such as the Comcáac, Seri, Tohono O'odham, and Yaqui, have incorporated this medicine into their practices. While some researchers and advocates have become vocal proponents of using only synthetic 5-MeO-DMT, it's crucial to recognize that such arguments can inadvertently discredit the traditional practices of the Sonoran Desert tribes.

The peoples of Sonora have a deep, symbiotic relationship with their land, which includes all the medicines and plants within their territory. Just as many Indigenous cultures evolve and adapt their practices over time, these tribes have thoughtfully integrated *el sapo* (the toad) into their existing medicine bag. We must be respectful of how we paint the picture in order to honor their practices with cultural sensitivity and respect for Indigenous sovereignty.

This area has been hard hit and impoverished for many generations. They now face the consequences of the "toad boom," including ecosystem damage from tourists and Mexican drug cartels. People drive around in 4x4s in search of toads, breaking up the desert's thin biofilm and harming the fragile ecosystem—home to the Arizona bark scorpion, the rare grasshopper mouse, and the Sonora mud turtle—which could potentially take decades to recover.

So, as many herpetologists and 5-MeO-DMT researchers say, "Leave the toads alone." Please don't harvest medicine on your own. Some herpetologists recommend letting local tribes do this harvesting, if any at all. Those who build relationships with local Sonoran tribes could potentially access the medicine in a humble and supportive way. While for others, opting for synthetic 5-MeO-DMT is a more sustainable alternative.

Legalities

The landscape of legality is shifting rapidly, yet many of these substances are still federally illegal in the United States. Other countries, such as Canada and Mexico, have more lax regulations that are substance specific. For example, 5-MeO-DMT is not currently regulated in Canada. Laws governing these substances vary by country and state, and even on a city level in the United States. Even within the states that have enacted decriminalization legislation, rules are outlined for personal use and how much a user can possess.

Some wrongful prosecutions have been overcome in the United States with legal support. There are even organizations in the psychedelic community that have funds to help people in specific situations. Obviously, selling psychedelics on Instagram is not one of them, as distribution outside of cannabis in licensed dispensaries is still strictly prohibited. Any substance that is considered Schedule 1 by the Drug Enforcement Administration (DEA) can lead users to face charges, even in municipalities that have decriminalized it on a local level. The chances are lower in jurisdictions where it is still in a legal grey area. Some recent cases have involved people receiving mail shipments of Schedule 1 plant substances that were intercepted, leading the receiver of the package to be arrested. Unless policy alters in the United States on a federal level, free use of psychoactive substances is not legal.

In 1993 a legal framework was established for ceremonial religious use of peyote for members of the Native American Church (NAC). Under the Religious Freedom Restoration Act (RFRA), other churches could be established for bona fide ceremonial religious use of San Pedro, ayahuasca, and psilocybin mushrooms. Anyone participating in psychedelic church ceremonies should understand that each individual branch requires RFRA approval, which typically involves a lawsuit. If a church has completed the proper legal filings, it can receive the designation but must follow certain rules of compliance. For instance, every RFRA church must have a formal membership and each member attending a ceremony must have a card confirming their membership. They must also have a DEA license and keep a log of every member, along with the dosage administered. The medicinal substance itself needs to be locked securely at two levels, in a locked room and in a locked case that only designated people can access. The substance must be from a DEA-approved source or else cultivated onsite. For instance, Santo Daime Church branches legally import their medicine from one source in Brazil. Anyone promoting or participating in ceremonies in a non-compliant church can face fines, imprisonment, and a potentially permanent mark on their criminal record. There are many pseudo churches, meaning they are not in compliance with regulatory requirements and legal filings, operating in the United States, and some have been raided. The most important issue evaluated in these cases is sincere use: whether the church is sincere in its religious practice. If the church doesn't comply with laws, the sincere use case is hard to prove.

I share this information having witnessed what has been happening in the psychedelic landscape over the last decade. I am in no way giving anyone legal advice, especially since laws can change and the grey areas are very grey, leaving them open for interpretation. It is imperative to know what legal risks you are taking when it comes to work with psychedelics and plant medicines and the only way to know for sure is to consult an attorney who specializes in this area. Many lawyers work in the cannabis space and can advise on other psychedelic substances—and attorney-client privilege protects your privacy.

At present, the only legal psychedelic therapy in the United States and in many international jurisdictions is ketamine therapy, although clinical therapeutic use of psilocybin and MDMA will likely soon be widely available in the United States and Canada. For someone with a life-threatening illness, under the Right to Try Act, one can also receive psychedelic therapy from any clinical provider doing research trials, as long as Phase 1 safety data has been completed. This means if you have a family member with a terminal illness who wants to have psychedelic therapy, they could reach out to one of the companies or groups running trials and request to receive treatment. You would have to pay out-of-pocket for the treatment, as insurance doesn't cover medications still being studied.

Legality is just one reason why I'll mainly focus here on the greater "work" of inner alchemy and seeding our consciousness. The plant medicine is simply a doorway to this—it's within a larger system that it brings transformation and the substances cannot do so by themselves. This is another reason why throughout the book I refer back to other modalities of entering altered states without psychedelics or plant medicines, such as holotropic breathwork, shamanic drumming, sound healing, flotation tanks, darkroom meditation, and other meditation practices. It's not illegal to get high on the endogenous DMT within your own body. In no way am I encouraging anyone to break any laws, even though I believe many of the laws are unfair, outdated and contradictory to the research data showing the profound benefits of therapeutic and psychospiritual work with plant medicine and psychedelics.

Gestational Stage

After presenting so much here, I will say—to prevent any confusion—that the information in this book is not intended as a substitute for proper training for administering psychedelic medicine, nor is it the purpose. Given the limited understanding of these topics in Western culture, it's important to emphasize that mastering these intricate knowledge systems requires extensive apprenticeship and community support to prioritize harm reduction and ensure a duty of care. The aim of this book, and this section in particular, is to offer guidance for your inner work amidst the rapid developments in the psychedelic sphere and to foster a renewed emphasis on respect, reciprocity, informed consent, and education. My intent is to serve as a guide to the expansive landscape of the evolving psychedelic movement, shedding light on its true origin, providing support for its responsible stewardship and make it a safe but profoundly transformative modality for healing.

There are also things I am not allowed to share here—as both a Bwiti initiate and due to many other privacy or legality issues caused by the current drug war in the United States and in other countries. As such, anything that may seem "missing" might be intentional. I have been rigorous in checking all quotes and information shared to make sure that permissions have been granted and information has been conveyed as accurately as possible. Taking these steps is essential, as we are still working in very delicate territory. Please know that I treat all of this information with the highest level of concern and respect for the well-being of all people, plants, and species.

Perhaps most of all, I want to convey the importance of slowing down and moving forward carefully, pausing frequently to check in on our direction and alignment. Because it's not how fast you go—it's how well you integrate what you've learned and experienced. Let's put the brakes on scaling up, for a bit, and let facilitators grow in their expertise, allow the proper spaces to be built, and focus on treating the whole person rather than some pathology. Let's step away from panaceas to do the real work that needs to be done. Let's lean into our collective pain and suffering. You have to feel it to heal it. Then, you might have to feel it again, and again, until you build your inner resilience.

Let's approach this gestational stage of movement with intelligence and compassion, taking the time to carefully design an infrastructure that serves the highest good rather than rushing in and risking avoidable errors. By learning to listen to and engage with these powerful tools thoughtfully, we can cultivate our own mastery from within. From this deeply embodied understanding, we can responsibly advance with these medicines, ensuring that traditional wisdom and its elders are honored with the respect and reverence they deserve.

I don't have all the answers to the many complex questions about plant medicines, but I do believe that if you picked up this book at this time in history, in some way you are a leader or pioneer or someone who has the potential to make a difference. And I believe the way forward is to create diverse councils of people invested in this work: elders, facilitators, therapists, traditional practitioners, and anyone who wants to learn collectively in a loving, non-self-serving space. We are in a fragile transition period of bridging worlds. But we're all in this together, learning how our global tribe can incorporate many generations' and continents' worth of ancestral healing into modern society. Thank you to all the elders and teachers who offered compassion and gentleness as I was learning and continue humbly to learn this walk.

I believe that even in chaos, nature will find order. As we make our way back into harmony with nature and connect with the web of life, we need to support one another, unify, and hold everyone accountable. We need our greater human tribe now more than ever. As they say in my Bwiti Fang family, *"Bi ne ayong da"*: "We are one clan."

Glossary

altered states of consciousness: these are any states that significantly differ from normal waking consciousness, often induced by practices like meditation, breathwork, or the use of psychoactive substances. These states can allow for unique perceptions, feelings, and thoughts.

Aluna: in Kogi Kággaba this term translates directly to "Moon," and is also applied to metaphysical concepts embodied by the celestial body. It is deeply connected to intuition and internal light.

ancestral DNA: refers to genetic material inherited from one's ancestors. It's the source of traits and conditions that can be traced through family lines.

ancestral healing: the process of healing ancestral traumas or wounds passed down through generations.

Ancestral Heart: Tricia Eastman's nonprofit organization focused on Indigenous-led biocultural preservation and reciprocity. "Ancestral Heart" is the collective voice of the ancestors.

ancestral trauma: refers to the trauma that has been passed down from previous generations.

ancient mystery school traditions: ancient teachings that revolve around esoteric wisdom and spiritual enlightenment, which were usually taught in secret schools where the knowledge was passed only to a select few who underwent certain initiatory rites. These teachings were often encoded in myths and allegories to protect their sacred knowledge. Examples of these traditions include the

Eleusinian Mysteries in ancient Greece, the Kemetic Mysteries of Isis and Osiris, and secret schools within the traditions of Hermeticism, Gnosticism, Kabbalah, and Rosicrucianism, among others.

archetype: symbolic, primal ideas or patterns of thought that reside in the unconscious, according to Swiss depth psychologist Carl Jung. They can be found in myth and fairy tales, religions, and spiritual traditions, and represent primal behaviors and experiences such as the archetype of the hero, the mother, or the trickster.

archetypal energies: universal symbols or patterns that are part of the collective unconscious, as theorized by Carl Jung. These energies manifest in our behavior, thoughts, and cultural symbols.

archetypal hero drive: a motivation rooted in the desire to be a savior or heroic figure, often influenced by colonialist narratives and cultural conditioning.

archetypal information: knowledge, characteristics, or patterns that are universally present and understood in the collective unconscious, often communicated through symbols or mythology.

archetypal realms: conceptual spaces occupied by archetypes, which are universal symbols or themes that have occurred across all cultures and epochs.

archetypal template: the set of archetypal influences, often interpreted through astrological signs, that shape an individual's personality, behaviors, tendencies, strengths, and weaknesses.

Arizona bark scorpion: a small, light brown scorpion commonly found in the Southwestern United States and Mexico. It is the most venomous scorpion in North America.

attachment: behavior that involves emotional dependence on another person or thing.

authentic traditional wisdom keeper: individual who has received proper initiation, training, and permission from a lineage or ancestral wisdom to administer plant medicines or engage in spiritual practices.

ayahuasca: a psychoactive brew used in traditional spiritual medicine in cultures of the Amazon basin. It's typically made from the vine *Banisteriopsis caapi* and the leaves of the *Psychotria viridis*. The brew, which contains N,N-Dimethyltryptamine or DMT (*see DMT*), is known for inducing altered states of consciousness that last for several hours.

Aztec: a Mesoamerican civilization that flourished in Central Mexico in the post-classic period from 1300 to 1521. The Aztec culture is generally grouped within the cultural complex known as the Nahuatl-speaking cultures, which includes the Toltec, Chichimec, and Teotihuacán civilizations.

banzi: a term in the Bwiti tradition that means "to hatch." It refers to someone who has undergone initiation in the Bwiti practice

Bardo: in Tibetan Buddhism it is the intermediate or transitional state between death and rebirth.

benben: a Kemetic term for the capstone of a pyramid or obelisk, symbolizing the primordial mound from which the Earth arose. In a cosmic sense, it represents the birthplace of light, similar to the singularity point.

bio-cultural heritage: the combined natural and cultural heritage of a region or community, including its biodiversity, ecosystems, and traditional knowledge.

biodynamic farming: an approach to agriculture that emphasizes the holistic interconnections within the farming system and incorporates both traditional methods and esoteric principles, including an emphasis on aligning farming activities with lunar cycles.

bioenergetic healing: healing methods that work with the energy systems of the body, such as the chakras and the aura. These methods often involve various forms of energy manipulation and visualization, with the goal of restoring balance and flow to the body's energy systems.

biopiracy: the unauthorized use, exploitation, or patenting of traditional knowledge, cultural practices, or biological resources from indigenous communities without their consent or fair compensation.

Black Moon Lilith: in astrology, this represents the apogee, or the furthest point of the Moon's orbit from the Earth. It governs our most primitive behaviors and is considered the "shadow" or hidden side of our nature.

Blessings of the Forest: a Gabonese organization involved in supporting local Bwiti villages in biocultural preservation and sustainable use of iboga.

blue lotus: an aquatic flower used in herbal medicine, often consumed as a tea. It is believed to have a relaxing and creativity-enhancing effect.

bridging worlds: connecting and integrating different perspectives, cultures, or realms of knowledge.

bruja: Spanish term for "witch." In the Latin American tradition, a bruja is a woman who practices witchcraft, typically involving magic, spell work, and healing.

Bwiti: a spiritual discipline primarily practiced by the forest-dwelling Babongo and Mitsogo peoples of Gabon (Central Africa) and by the Fang people of Gabon and Cameroon. Bwiti incorporates animism, ancestor worship, and insights drawn from experiences ingesting the African rootbark *Tabernanthe iboga*, which contains the psychedelic compound ibogaine.

Bwiti Fang: a branch of Bwiti and a spiritual path that includes the ritualistic use of the iboga plant for self-discovery, healing, and communication with ancestors.

Central Sun: in cosmological and metaphysical discourse, this term refers to a powerful, spiritual, or galactic source of energy at the center of the universe or galaxy. It's believed to influence spiritual evolution and consciousness. (*see Great Central Sun*)

ceremonial dreamwork: a ritualistic practice of sharing and interpreting dreams within a community, often facilitated by a spiritual guide. It serves as a tool for personal guidance and collective wisdom. (*see dreamwork*)

chakra system: a philosophical and physical model in Indian traditions that outlines seven or more "energy centers" or spiritual power points in the human body.

clairvoyance: the ability to gain information about an object, person, location, or physical event through extrasensory perception. Any person who is claimed to have such ability is said to be clairvoyant ("clear sighted").

collective unconscious: a term coined by Carl Jung, referring to structures of the unconscious mind shared among beings of the same species. It is proposed to be the reservoir of experiences and archetypal concepts shared universally.

commodification of traditions: the transformation of cultural practices or rituals into marketable products or experiences.

conscious action: deliberate actions taken with awareness and intention, aligned with one's mastery template and the soul's wisdom.

copalero: a copal resin burner in the Mēxica tradition that is consecrated through a special process of rituals performed around the moon cycles and other practices, which can last forty to fifty-two days.

corpus callosum: a large, C-shaped nerve fiber bundle found beneath the cerebral cortex in the brain that connects the left and right cerebral hemispheres and facilitates interhemispheric communication.

Corpus Hermeticum: a series of ancient Greek philosophical and religious texts, associated with the legendary philosopher Hermes Trismegistus. They deal with such topics as metaphysics, cosmology, alchemy, astrology, and spirituality. They point to the interconnectedness of all things.

cosmic order: the idea that the cosmos is arranged or functions according to a natural or divinely organized pattern or system, often believed to include cycles of evolution, death, and rebirth.

cosmic potential: the immense array of possibilities and knowledge contained within the cosmos, which we can access through inner exploration and communication with the spirit world.

cosmic unfolding: a concept referring to the ongoing, ever-evolving nature of the universe and its inherent processes.

cosmovision: a society's worldview that is shaped by cultural, historical, and philosophical factors. For example, the Kogi Kággaba people aim to end their lives "without debts," so they maintain balance with nature by making pagamentos (payments).

creative master: the aspect of ourselves that embodies our creative power and ability to manifest our desires.

cultural appreciation: an alternative approach that promotes care and respect when engaging with ancient lineages and cultural practices (as opposed to cultural appropriation, which refers to taking from another's tradition without respect or permission).

cultural authenticity: the quality of being genuine, respectful, and true to the cultural heritage and traditions being engaged with.

cultural mining: the act of extracting or exploiting elements of another culture without understanding or respect for their cultural significance.

cultural sensitivity: being aware and respectful of the cultural norms, values, and practices of others.

curanderismo: A traditional Latin American healing practice blending Indigenous Mesoamerican, European, and African influences. It uses medicinal plants and spiritual rituals, combining physical and spiritual approaches to healing.

death of the psyche: a phrase often used by Carl Jung, referring to the profound transformation of the psyche often associated with deep spiritual and psychological processes, including ego death.

default mode network: a network in the brain that is most active when a person is not focused on the outside world, during self-referential thought, daydreaming, or introspection. Psychedelics are known to affect the default mode network, often leading to changes in self-perception and thinking patterns.

dieta: a period of restricted diet and isolation used in curanderismo to establish a connection with a specific plant spirit or master plant.

dissolution of self: letting go of egoic identification and self-centered concerns to prioritize the needs of the community and greater whole.

divination: a practice that seeks to foretell future events or discover hidden knowledge through the interpretation of omens or by using supernatural powers. Common methods of divination include astrology, tarot card reading, rune casting, and the I Ching, among others.

DMT: dimethyltryptamine, a powerful psychedelic compound naturally produced in small amounts in the human brain, certain plants, and animals.

dreamwork: a method of accessing cosmic intelligence through analyzing and interpreting the symbols and messages that appear in our dreams. (*see ceremonial dreamwork*)

Druids: members of an ancient Celtic religious order that existed in Britain, Ireland, and Gaul.

duty of care: the responsibility to ensure the well-being and safety of others.

ecological sensitivity: the recognition that certain plants, particularly psychedelic plants, are ecologically sensitive and vulnerable to exploitation or extinction due to overharvesting or habitat destruction.

effulu: a ritual smoke bath in the Bwiti tradition, for which a smoke tent is created where an individual is fully enveloped for purification during initiation.

ego death: a state of loss or the disappearance of self-identity or individuated consciousness. It is a profound psychological event often encountered during intense experiences, such as psychedelic trips, spiritual experiences, or deep meditative states.

egoic template: the ego structure or ego identity that develops during early childhood. It serves as the blueprint that shapes how we experience and interact with the world. The egoic template often operates from the influences or "mirrors" in our environment, including our parents, societal institutions, media, and culture. It is also where unconscious behaviors are rooted.

electrochemical activation: a process that utilizes electrical energy to induce chemical reactions.

elemental fire: the transformative, destructive, and purifying aspect of nature.

embodiment: the process of integrating and living the principles, knowledge, or teachings of a certain tradition or body of knowledge fully and deeply—in the body. Unlike learning a skill through the mind, embodiment implies fully bringing the skill or teaching into your life in an embodied way.

Emerald Tablet: an ancient Hermetic text purportedly authored by Hermes Trismegistus, full of esoteric wisdom and principles, such as "as above, so below."

enneagram: a model of the human psyche that is principally understood and taught as a typology of nine interconnected personality types. It is used here as a tool for self-awareness and for understanding the shadow aspects of the ego.

Ensofic Ray (Ohr Ein Sof): Kabbalistic term referring to the initial, infinite light of Creation that illuminated the cosmos.

entheogens: chemical substances, typically of plant origin, which are ingested to produce a non-ordinary state of consciousness for religious or spiritual purposes. These substances are used in both modern and traditional contexts for spiritual growth, insight, healing, and the exploration of consciousness. Examples include psilocybin mushrooms, ayahuasca, and 5-MeO-DMT.

epigenetics: the study of changes in organisms caused by modification of gene expression rather than alteration of the genetic code itself.

Epigenetic research emphasizes the significant influence of ancestral experiences and early life interactions on the well-being of adult humans.

epigenetic tags: chemical modifications to DNA that do not change the sequence but can affect gene activity. These tags can be inherited and are responsible for some of the changes seen across generations. They can result from environmental influences and life experiences, including trauma.

extractive capitalist culture: a cultural and economic system that prioritizes profit and exploitation of natural resources, often at the expense of the environment and well-being of individuals and communities.

facilitator: a psychospiritual trained practitioner or psychedelic therapist who supports the process for the journeyer, providing guidance but not imposing their own ideas. They help in the integration of symbolic visions, prompt introspection through questions, and are trauma-informed in their approach.

feeling states: emotional states or conditions that we experience. These states can provide important insight into our internal reality and can serve as a form of nonverbal communication.

feminine principle: in spiritual and philosophical contexts, the feminine principle is associated with receptivity, creation, nurturing, compassion, understanding, and intuition. This is not tied to gender but is an integral part of the universal balance.

fiat currency: currency that has value because a government declares it to be legal tender, not because it is backed by a physical commodity like gold.

fractal nature of the cosmos: the idea that the structure of the universe is self-similar across different scales. Fractals are patterns that are invariant under scale transformations. This means they appear identical regardless of the level of magnification. When applied to the cosmos, this term suggests that similar patterns and geometric structures repeat at every scale, from the smallest subatomic particles to galaxies.

free will: the power to act independently of predetermined necessity or fate. In the context of soul kintsugi, free will is the ability to choose to lean inward, compassionately evolve, nurture oneself, and stay connected with one's soul.

GABA: short for Gamma-Aminobutyric Acid, a type of amino acid that acts as a neurotransmitter in the central nervous system and functions to promote relaxation and reduce stress by blocking and slowing down the speed at which information travels through the nervous system.

Graham Hancock: a British author known for his theories about ancient civilizations, Earth changes, stone monuments, or megaliths, altered states of consciousness, and ancient myths. The author of the book *Fingerprints of the Gods*, in which he lays out an argument for an advanced civilization that predates known history.

Great Central Sun: in metaphysical terms, this is considered the highest point of consciousness or intelligence, often equated with the concept of God or a Supreme Being. (*see Central Sun*)

harm reduction: policies, programs, and practices that aim to minimize negative health, social, and legal impacts associated with drug use, drug policies, and drug laws. Harm reduction is grounded in justice and human rights and focuses on positive change and working with people without judgment, coercion, discrimination, or requiring that they stop using drugs as a precondition of support.

healing arts: practices and modalities aimed at promoting healing and well-being, including traditional and alternative therapies.

Hermes Trismegistus: thought to be an ancient philosopher and prophet, considered the author of the *Corpus Hermeticum*. It's unclear whether he was a living historical figure or a god who was a syncretism of the Greek god Hermes and the Kemetic god Thoth.

hermetic principles: fundamental spiritual laws described in *The Kybalion*, a book of hermetic philosophy. The principles are attributed to Hermes Trismegistus. These principles are mentalism, correspondence, vibration, polarity, rhythm, cause and effect, and gender.

holotropic breathwork: a practice developed by Stanislav Grof that uses breathing techniques to facilitate access to non-ordinary states of consciousness, often for the purpose of self-exploration and healing.

hungry ghosts: a concept from Buddhism describing a state of constant craving or desire. Hungry ghosts are symbolic of individuals who seek validation and answers from external sources, manifesting in addictive or compulsive behaviors.

iboga: a perennial rainforest psychoactive shrub native to western Central Africa, traditionally used in spiritual and healing ceremonies. Bwiti practitioners consume its root bark to bring about intense visions and introspective experiences.

ibogaine: a naturally occurring psychoactive substance found in *Tabernanthe iboga*. It has been used traditionally by Indigenous African cultures and has been found to be effective in treating addictions.

imaginal realm: the mental space where images and symbols are born, often encountered in dreams or deep meditative states. It differs from imagination or the imaginary in that it doesn't refer to things humans "imagine"; instead, it represents an actual realm where aspects of the unseen reside.

inclusivity: the practice of including and embracing diverse perspectives, voices, and experiences.

Indigenous Peoples: as the original inhabitants of their respective regions, these communities hold unique cultural, historical, and ancestral ties to the lands they occupy. Their distinctive languages, traditions, spiritual beliefs, social structures, and lifestyles have been cultivated over centuries. However, these cultures have often grappled with significant adversities related to colonization, land dispossession, discrimination, and the preservation of their cultural heritage in the face of the encroaching pressures of Western ideologies.

Indigenous Peyote Conservation Initiative: an initiative dedicated to the preservation and conservation of peyote and its cultural significance.

individuated consciousness: a term referring to a state of consciousness in which the individual has developed a mature, integrated sense of self, distinct from the collective consciousness. This state involves having a deep understanding of the workings of the ego mind and being able to see beyond the limitations of the ego.

initiation: in the context of spiritual traditions, it refers to a rite of passage or a transformative experience that marks a person's transition into a new role, state, or level of understanding. It's often accompanied by rituals and practices designed to facilitate personal growth and transformation.

inner alchemy: a term from Jungian psychology referring to the process of self-transformation and self-realization, through which one integrates the various aspects of one's psyche.

inner critic: an internal voice that judges and diminishes one's self-worth. It is a concept used in psychology and psychotherapy to refer to a subpersonality that is judgmental and demeaning. The inner critic may push an individual to excel or perform in certain ways based on past conditioning.

inner eye: the mind's ability to visualize and perceive in the realm of our imagination. In spiritual terms, this can relate to the ability to receive visions or messages from the subconscious mind or spiritual realms.

inner moon: the inner self or soul, which is reflective and receptive, just as the Moon reflects the Sun's light. Connecting to your inner moon means observing and understanding your internal states and emotional landscape.

innerverse: the interior universe within each individual, often associated with personal consciousness, the psyche, or the soul. It mirrors the concept of the universe and emphasizes the interconnectedness of all things.

integration: the process of making sense of an experience (often profound or traumatic) and incorporating it into one's life and worldview. This is a key concept of psychology used in therapeutic processes involving transformative experiences, like psychedelic therapy.

integrity: acting in alignment with one's values, principles, and ethical standards.

interdependence: the reliance and interconnectedness of different beings and systems for mutual support and well-being.

Internal Family Systems (IFS): a therapeutic approach developed by American therapist Richard Schwartz.

International Center for Ethnobotanical Education, Research, and Service (ICEERS): an organization focused on the study and conservation of ethnobotanical knowledge.

intuitive hit: a sudden realization or understanding that arises from our intuition. Intuitive hits can provide important insights and guide us toward our true path.

journeyer: an individual undergoing a psychospiritual ceremony or a psychedelic therapeutic experience. They journey through their subconscious under the influence of the medicine, supported by a facilitator or therapist.

journeywork: a therapeutic practice of working with various techniques to address and heal the different "parts" of the ego that may be causing emotional dysregulation caused by trauma. Journeywork often involves the use of symbolic acts and rituals to engage with the subconscious mind, promoting healing and integration. This practice can be facilitated through psychedelic experiences, traditional indigenous ceremony, or therapeutic sessions.

Kabbalah: a tradition of Jewish mysticism that seeks to define the nature of the universe and the human being, the nature and purpose of existence, and various other ontological questions. Kabbalah uses classical Jewish sources to explain and demonstrate its esoteric teachings.

karma: a spiritual principle of cause and effect where intent and actions of an individual influence the future of that individual. Karma, as a concept, explains the transference of positive or negative experiences based on a person's actions in this life or previous ones.

Kemet: the native name of ancient Egypt. The term signifies the "Black Land" or "Land of the Black Soil," referring to the rich, fertile soil along the Nile River where the first settlements began.

Kemetic Mysteries: the spiritual practices, rituals, and belief systems of Kemet (ancient Egypt), often involving mythology, alchemy, and initiatory rites.

kintsugi: a Japanese art form in which broken pottery is repaired using gold to seal any cracks. The repaired item is considered more valuable than before it was broken. Used as a metaphor in the text, it refers to the process of healing and mending aspects of ourselves, emphasizing their increased value post-repair.

kundalini yoga: a form of yoga that involves the awakening of kundalini energy located at the base of the spine, involving chanting, breathwork, asana (postures), and meditation.

language of symbols: the method of communication used by the universe, in which each symbol has a unique vibrational frequency. This language extends beyond spoken or written words and includes a range of symbolism that speaks directly to our consciousness.

Law of Correspondence: the concept that the principles or laws of physics that explain the physical world, energy, light, vibration, and motion have their corresponding principles in the ether or universe: "as above, so below."

Law of Vibration: the idea that everything in the universe, regardless of its physical or non-physical nature, is in a state of constant vibration.

Legalize Nature: a movement advocating for the decriminalization and responsible use of natural entheogenic substances.

lineage keeper: See *wisdom keeper.*

lunar cycle: the cycle of phases that the moon goes through over about 29.5 days, from new moon to full moon and back to new moon.

lunar energy: symbolizes the feminine principle and governs the element of water. It represents rebirth, regeneration, introspection, emotions, intuition, and connection with the inner self.

lunar fast: a form of fasting associated with lunar energy, which includes consuming only water and light teas over a period of days. Its goal is to transcend desires, reset the body, and strengthen the immune system. It should only be done with medical or spiritual guidance.

lunar side: the intuitive and receptive aspect of ourselves associated with the Moon and feminine energy.

Māori: the Indigenous Polynesian people of New Zealand.

mastery template: the mental and spiritual framework that embodies one's highest potential and allows for the manifestation of authentic desires aligned with the soul's wisdom.

maternal source: the biological mother who nurtures and carries the baby in her womb. In a broader context, it can also mean any person or entity that provides sustenance, nurturing, or growth.

medicine drum: a traditional instrument used in various cultures for healing and spiritual ceremonies, believed to connect individuals with spiritual dimensions and natural rhythms.

medicine work: the process of self-healing and transformation facilitated by these substances, which are called medicines by many, often used in the context of plant medicine and psychedelic therapies.

meditation: a practice where an individual uses a technique, such as focusing their mind on a particular object, thought or activity, to achieve a mentally clarity and an emotionally calm and stable state.

mescaline: a naturally occurring psychedelic substance found in various cacti, including peyote and San Pedro.

microdosing: the practice of consuming small, sub-perceptual amounts of a psychoactive substance, such as psilocybin mushrooms, with the intention of promoting creativity, boosting performance, and enhancing cognitive function.

Moondance: A sacred annual rite for women performed by the Mēxica (descendants of the Aztecs). This ceremony is guided by the abuelas (grandmothers or female elders), who impart traditional teachings. The ritual's origins can be traced back to the *Borgia Codex*, an important pre-Columbian manuscript.

multidimensionaire: individual who can access and harness the infinite power of the universe to create the life they want, thereby being wealthy in ways beyond the material.

mycelium: the thread-like network of fungi that connects plants and trees in a forest, facilitating nutrient exchange and communication.

mycorrhizal network: a symbiotic association between fungi and plant roots, in which the fungi provide nutrients and aid in the absorption of water, contributing to the overall health and vitality of the plants.

mystical experience: an experience characterized by a sense of unity, transcendence of time and space, a deep sense of sacredness, and a sense of knowing the ultimate reality. This type of experience is often reported during deep meditation, prayer, near-death experiences, and the use of psychedelics.

mystical state: experience characterized by the loss of the usual sense of reality replaced by a sense of union with the divine or the universe.

nahual: in Mesoamerican folk religion, a nahual is a human being who has the power to shape-shift into an animal form, often after dark.

National Council of Native American Churches: an organization representing Native American churches and their religious practices.

neteru: the term used in Kemet for gods and goddesses. It implies beings who embody high potentials and qualities.

neurodivergent: a term that refers to individuals whose brains function differently from what is considered "typical." It includes conditions like ADHD, autism, dyslexia, etc.

Ngonde: "Moon" in the Bwiti tradition

nima: in the Bwiti tradition, these are individuals who perform initiations. They may undergo ten to fifteen years of training before they're given permission or handed the power to perform certain rituals related to the initiatic rites of a branch of Bwiti they represent.

non-attachment: a state of not giving any particular desire or outcome attention, allowing an individual to surrender to what is and approach life with curiosity. Non-attachment is key in meditation and the practice of presence, allowing for clearer reception of consciousness.

non-dual state: a state of consciousness in which the dichotomy between the self and the universe, or between the subject and the object, dissolves. It is often described as a state of unity or oneness, beyond the confines of the individual ego.

numinous: describing an experience that makes you fearful yet fascinated, awed yet attracted—the powerful, personal feeling of being overwhelmed and inspired. It refers to the experience of transcendent or divine power.

okoume trees: a species of tree native to the forests of Gabon and used in the Bwiti tradition, known for the medicinal properties of its resin and for its traditional use in spiritual ceremonies.

Original Peoples: the indigenous or native inhabitants of a specific land or region. (*see Indigenous Peoples*)

pagamento: offering made by the Kogi Kággaba, often in cotton, which represent a payment back to Creator for the things they utilize from nature.

paternal care: caregiving that typically embodies strength, provision, and protection, traditionally associated with masculine energies. A lack of balanced paternal care can contribute to unhealthy ego formation and related behavioral issues.

peptide: short chains of amino acids, the building blocks of proteins, which play vital roles in biological functions.

perinatal matrix: a concept in transpersonal psychology that describes the four-stage process of birth and its profound psychological impact on an individual.

pharmaceutical feedstock: raw materials or substances used in the production of pharmaceutical drugs.

piezoelectric energy: a type of energy that results from pressure or heat. In the context of spiritual practices, this energy is believed to enhance our ability to access deeper states of consciousness, intuition, and spiritual insight. This term is often associated with the calcite microcrystals found in the pineal gland.

pineal gland: also known as the epiphysis cerebri, it's a small endocrine gland in the brain of most vertebrates. The pineal gland produces melatonin, serotonin, and other biochemical substances, and is believed to play a role in regulating sleep and dream cycles. In spiritual traditions, it is often associated with intuition and spiritual insight.

plant medicine: the use of plants and their extracts to heal and holistically address overall wellness, often based on traditional knowledge and practices. Some of these plants contain psychoactive compounds that, when used ceremonially, can induce altered states of consciousness.

popoxcomitl: (*see copalero*)

presence: the state of being fully engaged and attentive to the present moment, without being lost in thoughts or distractions.

prima materia: in alchemical teachings, translating to "first substance." It refers to the purest and greatest expression of our true potential to manifest reality. Prima materia is associated with creative energy that flows when we are present and open to new possibilities.

principle of gender: an ancient hermetic concept from the alchemical text *The Kybalion*, positing that both masculine and feminine qualities are present in everything. These complementary aspects work together to create balance and harmony.

Prometheus: in Greek mythology, the Titan who stole fire from the gods and gave it to humans. This act brought humans knowledge and progress but also invited the wrath of the gods.

psilocybin: a naturally occurring psychedelic compound produced by more than two hundred species of mushrooms. The compound, belonging to a class of substances known as tryptamines, can induce profound changes in consciousness marked by alterations in sensory perception, thought processes, and a heightened state of awareness.

psyche: the human soul, mind, or spirit. It represents the mental or psychological structure of a person, especially as a motivating force.

psychedelic initiations: ceremonial or structured experiences using psychedelic substances, typically for the purpose of spiritual growth or personal transformation.

psychedelics: psychoactive substances often used to assist in personal transformation, growth, and the cultivation of deeper connections with life. They can help quiet the ego, bring awareness to neglected aspects of self, and promote a sense of interbeing or unity with all things.

psychedelic therapy: the therapeutic use of psychedelic substances, often in a controlled and supportive setting, to facilitate psychological healing and personal growth.

psychedelic tourism: traveling to specific destinations to participate in psychedelic experiences or ceremonies.

psychoactive substances: substances that have significant effects on mental processes. These can include plant medicines, synthetic drugs, and certain types of fungi. They are often used in religious or spiritual contexts to induce altered states of consciousness.

psychomagic: a term popularized by Chilean film director Alejandro Jodorowsky involving the use of initiatory rituals to heal psychospiritual wounds.

purgatory plants: psychoactive plants or substances that induce purging, such as vomiting or cleansing of the body, as part of purification rituals in certain traditions.

purge: the process of releasing and letting go of elements of trauma, often physically such as vomiting, emotionally such as crying, or mentally such as experiencing certain memories that come up to be processed. These types of purges center around transformative experiences such as during a psychedelic journey, intense meditation, breathwork, or trauma release.

quantum consciousness: a theory proposing that consciousness is deeply linked to the fundamental workings of the quantum universe.

reagents: substances used in a chemical reaction to detect, measure, or produce other substances

reciprocity: the practice of giving back, exchanging, or sharing in a mutually beneficial way.

Religious Freedom Restoration Act (RFRA): a U.S. federal law that protects religious freedom and allows individuals and groups to exercise their religious beliefs without interference from the government.

rematriate: the act of returning or restoring land, resources, or cultural heritage to Indigenous communities, often emphasizing the role of women in this process.

right relationship: the harmonious and respectful connection between humans, nature, and spiritual practices.

sacrament: a religious or spiritual ritual believed to impart mystical blessings, often involving symbolic actions or substances, some of which may induce altered states through psychoactive compounds or plants.

scarcity: a mindset characterized by a fear of lack and limited resources, leading to a sense of competition and hoarding.

Schedule 1: a classification of substances under the U.S. Controlled Substances Act indicating a high potential for abuse and no accepted medical use.

schism of the soul: describes a state of disconnection from one's soul, often manifesting as a lack of joy, feelings of meaninglessness, or creative blockage. This disconnection is believed to cause various mental and emotional disorders.

seeding consciousness: the practice of planting intention and awareness to initiate positive change and transformation.

sequoia: a species of tree known for its massive size and long life. It serves as a metaphor in this text for resilience and rebirth after devastation.

Seri: an Indigenous tribe native to the Sonoran Desert region.

serotonin: a neurotransmitter that contributes to feelings of well-being and happiness. It also plays a role in regulating mood, social behavior, appetite, sleep, memory, and sexual desire and function.

serpent path: a term used in various spiritual traditions, referring to the path of spiritual ascent, symbolized by a serpent or snake.

set and setting: a foundational principle in psychedelic experiences that emphasizes the importance of creating a safe and supportive environment (setting) and being in the right mindset (set) to maximize the potential benefits and minimize risks.

shadow: a term from Carl Jung's analytical psychology, referring to the unconscious.

singularity point: a concept in cosmology referring to a point of infinite density where the laws of physics break down. Often equated with black holes in modern physics, it also has metaphysical interpretations, including a connection to the highest source of consciousness or light.

solar power: an analogy to describe the active, conscious mind, often associated with productivity and materialistic ideals in Western societies.

somatic bodywork: a therapeutic technique that involves hands-on manipulation of the body, with the aim of improving bodily awareness and addressing physical issues related to stress and trauma carried in the body.

soul kintsugi: a process of soul retrieval or reintegration, in which broken or disconnected aspects of the self are "glued" back together, often through the use of initiatic rites or psychoactive substances. The result is a self that is more valuable and more whole than before. (*see kintsugi*)

soul reclamation: the process of healing and reintegrating parts of the self that may seem broken or out of sorts. It's a metaphor for personal growth and self-improvement, often through the means of psychotherapy or spiritual practices. This term draws on the metaphor of kintsugi, a Japanese art form that repairs broken pottery with gold, thereby enhancing its value.

sovereignty: the power and authority to govern oneself and make independent choices.

spiritual protocols: rituals, practices, and guidelines established by indigenous communities to ensure respectful ettiquette in engaging with the spirit world, its guardians, and spiritual traditions.

stewardship: the responsible management and care of something, such as land, resources, or cultural traditions, to ensure their preservation and sustainability.

surrender: the act of letting go of resistance and control, allowing life's circumstances to unfold and trusting in the wisdom of the universe.

survivalist programming: the instinctual and often subconscious patterns of behavior and thought that are created to ensure survival during childhood. These patterns can be problematic when they become overactive or inappropriate to the current environment or situation.

synchronicities: meaningful coincidences that appear in our lives as a sign or message from the universe. Interpreting synchronicities can provide guidance and insight regarding our path forward.

synthetic drugs: pharmaceuticals or substances produced artificially through chemical synthesis.

Tabernanthe iboga: (*see iboga*)

tantra: a genre of ancient Indian texts that discuss various esoteric practices. In the Western world, "tantra" is often misconstrued to be an exclusively sexual practice, but it has more to do with spiritual practices and concepts aimed at channeling cosmic energies to awaken the divine essence within the individual.

third eye: in Eastern spiritual traditions, the third eye is a metaphorical inner eye or sense that represents enlightenment and the ability to perceive beyond ordinary sight. It's often associated with visions, intuition, and the ability to recognize subtle energies.

Tohono O'odham: an Indigenous tribe native to the Sonoran Desert.

traditional wisdom: knowledge and practices passed down through generations within a specific culture or tradition.

transcendent function: a concept from Carl Jung's analytical psychology. The transcendent function arises when an individual faces a psychological conflict or tension between two opposing forces or complexes. The emergence of a third, unifying element leads to personal growth and integration.

transpersonal psychology: a subfield of psychology that integrates spiritual and transcendent aspects of the human experience within the framework of modern psychology.

trauma release: the process of identifying, processing, and releasing trauma from the body and mind. This can be facilitated by a variety of therapeutic approaches, including psychotherapy, bodywork, and psychedelic therapy.

tune in: a process that involves grounding ourselves and finding presence, allowing us to listen and trust the information we receive during intuitive sessions by our intention, or by focusing on or communicating with our inner knowing. This practice aims to let the full message be revealed without rushing to make sense of it.

Instead we allow the pieces to unveil themselves and slowly integrate them into a greater understanding of the parts at play in a situation, or when looking for direction toward the highest and best possible outcome.

unconscious: aspects of mental processes that occur without conscious awareness, such as automatic thoughts, feelings, or desires.

unitive consciousness: a state of consciousness in which a person feels a sense of unity or interconnectedness with all things. This is often reported during deep meditation, mystical experiences, and psychedelic journeys.

universal life force energy: a concept found in several spiritual and healing practices such as tai chi and qigong, it refers to the energy, sometimes referred to as chi or prana, that sustains all living beings.

urushi: a Japanese lacquer made from tree sap, which takes weeks to set. It is used in the traditional kintsugi process and serves as a metaphor in soul kintsugi for the time, patience, and care needed to heal the soul.

Vedism: the oldest stratum of religious activity in India for which there exist written materials. Knowledge of Vedic religion is derived from these surviving texts and also from certain rites that continue to be observed within the framework of modern Hinduism.

vision interpretation: the process of understanding and finding meaning in the symbols and messages received during visionary experiences, such as those induced by psychedelic journeys or deep meditations.

vision quest: a rite of passage observed among the Mēxica peoples and in many North American Indigenous traditions, in which an initiate abstains from food and water for several days while sitting in isolation in the wilderness. This practice, often accompanied by sacred fires and songs, is believed to induce mystical visionary experiences.

void: a state of complete emptiness or nothingness frequently encountered in deep meditation or during intense psychedelic experiences.

It's often described as a state of complete peace, beyond the confines of individual consciousness.

wabi sabi: a Japanese concept that finds beauty in imperfection and accepts the natural cycle of growth and decay. It is an aesthetic worldview that encourages acceptance of transience and imperfection.

web of life: the interconnectedness and interdependence of all living beings and the natural world.

Yaqui: an Indigenous tribe native to the Sonoran Desert region.

yin yoga: a slow-paced style of yoga in which poses are held for longer periods of time. This type of yoga is often beneficial for stress release and deep tissue stretching.

Zheti-ata: a tradition in the Kazakh culture that honors the spirits of seven generations of ancestors, preserved despite centuries of regional change and outside influences. The Kazakh people, historically nomadic, inhabit Kazakhstan and neighboring countries in Central Asia.

Bibliography

Because hyperlinks do not always remain viable, we are no longer including URLs in our resources, notes, or bibliographic entries. Instead we are providing the name of the website where this information may be found.

Abd El-Aziz, Tarek Mohamed, Yucheng Xiao, Jake Kline, Harold Gridley, Alyse Heaston, Klaus D. Linse, Micaiah J. Ward, Darin R. Rokyta, James D. Stockand, Theodore R. Cummins, Luca Fornelli, and Ashlee H. Rowe. "Identification and Characterization of Novel Proteins from Arizona Bark Scorpion Venom That Inhibit Nav1.8, a Voltage-Gated Sodium Channel Regulator of Pain Signaling." *Toxins* 13, no. 7 (July 2021): 501.

Acosta-Urquidi, Juan. "QEEG Studies of the Acute Effects of the Visionary Tryptamine DMT." *Cosmos and History: The Journal of Natural and Social Philosophy* 11, no. 2 (November 2015): 115–29.

Aristotle, and Richard McKeon. *The Basic Works of Aristotle.* New York: Random House, 1941.

Artemidorus, and Martin Hammond, *The Interpretation of Dreams.* Edited by Peter Thonemann. UK: Oxford University Press, 2020.

Baconnier, Simon, Sidney B. Lang, Maria Polomska, Bozena Hilczer, Garry Berkovic, and Guilia Meshulam. "Calcite Microcrystals in the Pineal Gland of the Human Brain: First Physical and Chemical Studies." *Bioelectromagnetics* 23, no. 7 (October 2002): 488–95.

Caird, Dale. "The Structure of Hood's Mysticism Scale: A Factor-Analytic Study." *Journal for the Scientific Study of Religion* 27, no. 1 (March 1988): 122–27.

Callaway, J. C. "Tryptamines, Beta-Carbolines and You." *Newsletter of the Multidisciplinary Association for Psychedelic Studies (MAPS)* 4, no. 2.

Cameron, Layne. "Mighty Mouse Uses Scorpion Venom as Painkiller." MSUToday (website). October 24, 2013. Accessed July 14, 2023.

Chia, Mantak. *Darkness Technology*. Universal Tao Publications, 2002.

Dass, Ram. *Remember, Be Here Now*. San Cristobal, NM: Lama Foundation, 1971.

Dixon, Jana. *Biology of Kundalini: Exploring the Fire of Life*. Boulder, CO: Emancipation Unlimited LLC, 2020.

Dobbs, David. "Zen Gamma." *Scientific American* (website), April 1, 2005, 9.

Duhm, Dieter. *The Sacred Matrix: From the Matrix of Violence to the Matrix of Life, The Foundation for a New Civilisation*. Frankfurt: Verlag Meiga, 2001.

Edinger, Edward F., and Joan Dexter Blackmer. *The Mystery of the Coniunctio: Alchemical Image of Individuation*. Toronto: Inner City Books, 1994.

Eliade, Mircea, "Inner Alchemy," in *Parabola: Myth and the Quest for Meaning*, edited by D. M. Dooling, vol. 3, no. 3, Madison, WI: Tamarack Press, 1978.

Evans-Wentz, W. Y. *The Tibetan Book of the Dead*. Princeton: Princeton University Press, 1927.

Gadalla, Moustafa. *Egyptian Cosmology: The Animated Universe*. Greensboro, NC: Tehuti Research Foundation, 2022.

Grof, Stanislav. 1998. "Human Nature and the Nature of Reality: Conceptual Challenges from Consciousness Research." *Journal of Psychoactive Drugs* 30, no. 4 (September 2011): 343–57.

Hall, Manly P. *The Secret Teachings of All Ages: An Encyclopedic Outline of Masonic, Hermetic, Qabbalistic and Rosicrucian Symbolical Philosophy*. Los Angeles: Philosophical Research Society, 1975.

Hameroff, Stuart. "Quantum Computation in Brain Microtubules? The Penrose–Hameroff 'Orch OR' Model of Consciousness." *Philosophical Transactions of the Royal Society A* 356, no. 1743 (August 1998): 1869–96.

Hesser, Jessica. "Read." Jessica Alix Hesser (website). Accessed July 13, 2023.

Huxley, T. H. "Nature: Aphorisms by Goethe." *Nature* 1 (1869): 9–11.

Jivanmukti. *Invoking Reality: The Spontaneous Teachings of Jivanmukti on the Essence of Spiritual Awakening & Siddha Kundalini Yoga*. Edited by J. Henry, P. Walters, and C. Edward. Jivanmukti & Siddhantha Yoga Academy, 2021.

Jodorowsky, Alejandro. *Psychomagic: The Transformative Power of Shamanic Psychotherapy*. Rochester, VT: Inner Traditions, 2010.

Jung, Carl G. *The Transcendent Function*. Zurich: The Student's Association of the C. G. Jung Institute, 1957.

Lao Tzu, *Tao Te Ching: The New Translation from Tao Te Ching: The Definitive Edition*. trans. Jonothan Star. New York: Jeremy P. Tarcher/Penguin, 2008.

Liddell, Henry George, and Robert Scott. *A Greek-English Lexicon: Compiled by Henry George Liddell and Robert Scott: A New Edition Revised and Augmented throughout by Henry Stuart Jones*. Oxford: Clarendon Press, 1948.

Men, Weiwei, Dean Falk, Tao Sun, Weibo Chen, Jianqi Li, Dazhi Yin, Lili Zang, and Mingxia Fan. "The Corpus Callosum of Albert Einstein's Brain: Another Clue to His High Intelligence?" *Brain* 137, no. 4 (April 2014): e268.

Miller, Jenesse. "Cycles of a Fasting-Mimicking Diet Help Mice Live Longer, Healthier." USC Leonard Davis School of Gerontology (website), October 14, 2021. Accessed July 14, 2023.

Ñāṇamoli, Bhikkhu, and Bhikkhu Bodhi, trans. "Latukikopama Sutta: Sutta 66" in *The Middle Length Discourses of the Buddha: A Translation of the Majjhima Nikāya*. Boston: Wisdom Publications, 1995 538-44.

Ñāṇamoli, Bhikkhu, and Bhikkhu Bodhi, trans. "Sunakkhatta Sutta: Sutta 105" in *The Middle Length Discourses of the Buddha: A Translation of the Majjhima Nikāya*. Boston: Wisdom Publications, 1995 868-74.

Nonnos. *Dionysiaca*, vol. III. W.H.D. Rouse (Cambridge, MA: Harvard University Press, 1940), 44:226–29.

Parry, Bruce, created by *Tribe, Penan*. Season 3, episode 6. Aired September 24, 2013, on BBC.

Robertson, John. "Flight Instructions for Psilocybin Journeys: Bill Richards." Maps of the Mind (website). August 26, 2020.

Santini, Céline. *Kintsugi: Finding Strength in Imperfection*. Kansas City: Andrews McMeel Publishing, 2019.

Scarre, Christopher. *Human Past: World Prehistory and the Development of Human Societies*. London: Thames & Hudson, 2013.

Schwartz, Richard C., and Martha Sweezy. *Internal Family Systems Therapy*. 2nd ed. New York: The Guilford Press, 2019.

Sherriff, Lucy. "Scientists in China Discover Rare Moon Crystal That Could Power Earth." Discovery (website). Accessed on October 15th, 2022.

Silva, Freddy. *The Divine Blueprint: Temples, Power Places, and the Global Plan to Shape the Human Soul*. n.p.: Invisible Temple, 2012.

Simonsson, Otto, José Carlos Bouso, Florian Kurth, Dráulio B. Araújo, Christian Gaser, Jordi Riba, and Eileen Luders. "Preliminary Evidence of Links between Ayahuasca Use and the Corpus Callosum." *Frontiers in Psychiatry* 13 (October 2022): 1002455.

Swan, John. *The Speculum Mundi*. Cambridge: Printed by the Printers to the Universitie of Cambridge, 1643.

Tarnas, Richard. *Cosmos and Psyche: Intimations of a New World View*. New York: Plume, 2007.

Walsch, Neale Donald. *Conversations with God, Book 3: Embracing the Love of the Universe*. Charlottesville, VA: Hampton Roads Publishing Company, 2020.

Index